Psychology in Vision Care

To my mother, Audrey Smith. She did not live to see this book completed, but her memory remains a great source of inspiration and encouragement.

Psychology in Vision Care

Rosalyn H. Shute BSc, PhD, AFBPsS, C. Psychol.
Discipline of Psychology
School of Social Sciences
The Flinders University of South Australia
Australia

formerly at

Department of Optometry
University of Wales College of Cardiff
UK

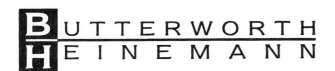

Butterworth-Heinemann Ltd
Linacre House, Jordan Hill, Oxford OX2 8DP

 PART OF REED INTERNATIONAL BOOKS

OXFORD LONDON BOSTON
MUNICH NEW DELHI SINGAPORE SYDNEY
TOKYO TORONTO WELLINGTON

First published 1991

© Butterworth-Heinemann Ltd 1991

British Library Cataloguing in Publication Data
Shute, Rosalyn H.
  Psychology in vision care.
  I. Title
  617.7

ISBN 0 7506 1417 X

Composition by Scribe Design, Gillingham, Kent
Printed and bound in Great Britain by Clays Ltd, St. Ives, plc.

Contents

Preface

For 2½ years, I worked as the only psychologist in the University of Wales College of Cardiff's Department of Optometry. It was a great learning experience: I attended a departmental course on optometry for medics, and learned about optometry 'on the job' through involvement in clinical and research work, conferences and seminars.

Having previous research experience with children (in educationally related research), my primary tasks were to participate in a project on the development of optokinetic nystagmus in children with strabismus, and to act as a consultant for child patients with reading problems. However, I became a psychological Jill-of-all-trades, never knowing from one day to the next which other areas of knowledge colleagues and students would ask me to draw upon. They sought advice about topics as diverse as experimental design and statistics, questionnaire preparation, dyslexia, developmental disabilities, stress and the effects of strokes. On a more formal basis, I introduced undergraduate lectures on communicating with patients, including young children and those with special needs, as well as supervising student projects.

Within the Visual Assessment Unit, in addition to assisting with the vision testing of infants, I was consulted about patients with special needs: these included people with disabilities caused by brain injuries and intellectual impairment, as well as children with learning difficulties. I also gave seminars on such topics as the development of premature babies and those with Down's syndrome.

My experience in the department convinced me of the great relevance of psychology to clinical optometry, yet the interface between the two disciplines is not well developed in comparison with the relationship between psychology and other medical and paramedical professions. That is what prompted me to write this volume. In it, I offer some useful ideas from psychology which have, as yet, barely percolated through to the optometric community, and hope that the book may act as a catalyst for further work in the area. I have tried to do justice to both optometric and psychological science while retaining readability; I have aimed to provide sufficient referencing to support the text without becoming turgid. I have also tried to maintain a practical approach throughout, drawing upon clinical experience as well as published literature and making explicit the connections between the psychological topics under consideration and clinical practice.

However, this is not a handbook of vision testing—it would be arrogant for a psychologist to write such a book!—although various tests and procedures are mentioned at various points. A basic knowledge of the visual system and vision testing is assumed. Although the book was written mainly for practising optometrists and students and teachers of optometry, it should also be of interest to others involved in vision care, such as ophthalmologists, orthoptists and ophthalmic nurses, as well as students of those subjects.

There are many people without whose direct or indirect input this book could not have been written. First and foremost are the optometrists with whom I have had the pleasure of working most closely in the Visual Assessment Unit: Margaret Woodhouse (its Director and powerhouse), Carol Westall (who was brave enough to share her research and her office with a psychologist) and Susan Leat, with her expertise on low vision. I thank all of them, and also Nick Rumney of the Low Vision Clinic, for offering helpful comments on the first draft of the book. Other colleagues in the department, headed firstly by Michel Millodot and latterly by Stuart Hodson, have also helped to create a pleasant and collaborative working atmosphere. I must also thank Geoff Nuttall, formerly of Butterworths, who was instrumental in getting my ideas off the ground, and his colleagues at Butterworth-Heinemann, who were persuaded that it was a good idea to produce an optometry book which was rather different in approach from their usual publications. Finally, I must thank my husband Jason, children Steffan and Elen and mother-in-law Mag, firstly for not complaining too much when I spent too long at my word-processor, and secondly, for being prepared to follow me in my forthcoming move from Cardiff to the Discipline of Psychology, The Flinders University of South Australia, Adelaide. I should be very pleased to hear from any readers who would like to contact me there.

Rosalyn H. Shute
November, 1990

Chapter 1

The nature of psychology

Introduction

A psychologist who leaves the safe confines of his or her own discipline is likely to meet two diametrically opposed reactions. On the one hand are those within other professions who display a keen interest in finding out what psychology can offer, and a scan of the popular optometry journals reveals a good degree of interest in the application of psychology to vision care. For example, Roberts (1988) has discussed the psychology of fitting rigid gas permeable lenses, Legerton (1989) has written about the importance of being a 'personable' practitioner and I was myself invited to write an article about patient anxiety (Shute, 1986).

On the other hand, however, there are those who regard psychology with deep suspicion. Practitioners working in science-based disciplines in particular sometimes resent those who attempt to invade their professional territory armed with what may be perceived as unscientific mumbo-jumbo.

Such scepticism is often based on ignorance of the true nature of psychology, and the discipline has to fight hard to convey a more accurate image than is often portrayed. This can be an uphill battle, as illustrated by the response of one journalist to a media release about an international conference on practical aspects of memory. The journalist telephoned to enquire whether any of the delegates had lost their way to the venue. Clearly, a 'Psychologist Forgets Way to Memory Conference' story was regarded as more news-worthy than an item on the contribution of psychology to our understanding of Alzheimer's disease, to promoting better learning in schoolchildren or to ensuring that a patient will remember vital medical information after a consultation. Psychology is always good for a laugh, and its frequent misportrayal in the past is one reason why books aimed at other professions almost invariably begin with an explanation of what psychology is really about. This one is no exception. This introductory chapter is aimed at dispelling some of the myths that continue to surround it, and also at outlining why

some of the most recent developments mean that the time is ripe
for a consideration of the ways in which psychology can enhance
vision care.

The subject matter of psychology

Despite the best educational efforts of the profession, the nature of
psychology still appears to be a matter for some confusion amongst
the general public. Those of us who are psychologists have learned
to be careful of when and how to admit to our calling. There is a
persisting belief that psychology is about lying on a couch and
revealing your inner self, and new acquaintances tend either to
shrink (sic) in horror in case you psychoanalyse them, or to corner
you and regale you with their personal problems. Alternatively,
psychologists are seen as people in white coats who know a great
deal about the behaviour of laboratory rats but are very remote
from the real world. Both myths have truthful roots in the history
of the discipline, but paint a very distorted picture of modern
psychology. Let us first examine these two erroneous stereotypes
before going on to consider the true nature of psychology today.

Psychology is frequently confused with psychiatry and psychoanalysis. Psychiatry is a specialist branch of medicine concerned with
psychiatric illness, and drugs are frequently a component of treatment.
Psychoanalysis is a form of psychotherapy based on Freudian theory;
confusingly, it is practised both by certain psychiatrists and by some
therapists who are not medically qualified. Freud, who was a medical
man, contributed a great deal to the development of both psychiatry
and psychology, particularly in drawing attention to the importance
of subconscious processes and of the early years of life. However,
the scientific basis of his work is highly questionable (Farrell, 1963).
Relatively few psychologists today would consider Freudian theory
an adequate basis for the treatment of psychological problems. Those
involved in such work—usually clinical psychologists—use a range
of other methods, including various forms of 'talking therapy', and
do not prescribe drugs.

The other stereotype, of the psychologist cloistered in an ivory
tower with white rats, arises from the behaviourist tradition
prevalent in the 1950s. It was argued that what went on in people's
minds was not open to scientific scrutiny. Only what they did or said
(their behaviour, including their verbal behaviour) was observable,
and therefore a legitimate object for investigation. It is true that a
great deal of 'rat work' went on at that time, aimed at developing
general principles of behaviour. This approach still has its advocates, and behaviourist principles remain influential, particularly in
the area of behaviour therapy and, as will be seen in later chapters,

there are instances where behavioural techniques are useful in clinical optometry. However, within psychology, other approaches have taken their place alongside behaviourism, and the study of animal behaviour has become increasingly divorced from mainstream psychology.

The definition of psychology which I favour is 'the scientific study of behaviour and experience'. Others may have their own variations of this, depending on their own particular viewpoint. Some might include the word 'human', wishing explicitly to exclude work on animal behaviour; however, my view is that we should retain the possibility that studying animals will sometimes help us to understand human behaviour, just as much of our understanding of the visual system has been based on animal models. The inclusion of the word 'experience' is indicative of the swing away from strict behaviourism. Thoughts and feelings, which are exactly what many lay people imagine psychology to be about, have once again become a respectable aspect of the subject, worthy of scientific attention.

There is another possible reason why the public may be confused about the nature of psychology, and that is the very ubiquity of the subject. Psychology has a relevance to any field of human endeavour. It is about what people feel, think and do and why they do it; how they learn, how they relate to one another and to their environment; how they interact with machines or operate within organizations. Psychological investigations can concentrate on individuals or on groups; they can focus in on physiology or pan out to the level of culture. The field is so vast that psychology graduates who wish to pursue the subject professionally (and now, in the UK, to become chartered psychologists) must undertake further specialist training which fits them for their chosen field, whether clinical, educational, occupational (industrial) or academic work. Thus although all psychologists share a certain basis of knowledge and understanding and are bound by the same ethical codes of conduct within their national professional organizations (such as the British Psychological Society and the American Psychological Association), they cannot easily step into one another's shoes, any more than a general practitioner and a brain surgeon could swap roles.

Psychology and health

This growing diversity and specialization within the subject is perhaps inevitable and not in itself undesirable, but this trend does need to be counterbalanced by a synthesizing force if psychologists are not to lose sight of relevant advances in areas other than their own. Paradoxically, perhaps, the development over the past few years of a new specialism, the field of health psychology, is providing one such integrative force. Health psychology is concerned not just with mental health, in the tradition of clinical psychology, but also with physical health (Johnston, 1990). In reality, the mental/ physical dichotomy is a false one, and health psychology is very much concerned with the inter-relationships between so-called 'mental' (or behavioural) and 'physical' aspects of health and illness.

One very important change in health care which health psychology is helping to bring about is the move away from a medical model towards a biopsychosocial approach to health and illness. The medical approach, which still holds sway overall, conceptualizes illness as resulting from a disorder within an individual's body, to be cured by interventions such as medication and surgery. This view is certainly an improvement over earlier notions that illness resulted from evil forces, but it is too limited. As its name indicates, the biopsychosocial approach recognizes that health and illness cannot be understood without considering the interactions between biological, psychological and social factors. Increasing emphasis is therefore being put on environmental and behavioural factors relevant for the promotion of good health and the prevention and and management of illness (Shute and Penny, 1989).

Many traditional areas of psychology have something to offer in increasing our understanding of health-related behaviour. For example, social psychology can promote understanding of the effects of attitudes towards health on the take-up of health care services. It can also cast light on problems of patient–practitioner communication. Another example is afforded by developmental psychology, which can offer insights into children's health-related behaviour and understanding at different ages—vital knowledge for health care professionals who work with children (Wilkinson, 1988).

The recent growth in health-related psychological knowledge means that there now exists a body of information of great potential benefit for vision care, although optometry does appear to have largely escaped the notice of psychologists as a profession worthy of study in itself. In keeping with the eclectic nature of health psychology, this book draws together relevant psychological knowledge from a wide range of areas. Its aim is to offer, for the enrichment of vision care, insights and practical suggestions derived from psychological science. To dispel any lingering suspicions that such knowledge is simply common sense, or the result of armchair philosophizing, the status of psychology as a science will be discussed before moving on to consider specifically its relationship with optometry.

Psychology as a science

Science and common sense

The majority of psychologists regard their discipline as a science. It seems reasonable, therefore, to begin by asking what it is that makes an area of endeavour classifiable as such, and we need to turn to philosophy to address this question. At one time, scientific enquiry took the form of observing and experimenting, and deriving general laws from one's observations. However, a change in emphasis has occurred during the 20th century, the views of the late Sir Karl Popper (in Mace, 1957) have been particularly influential. His view was that experimentation and observation should be driven by theory. However, he maintained that a theory can never be finally proved, only disproved, and when evidence against it is found the theory must be modified—this process represents scientific progress. According to Popper, if one cannot make refutable predictions from one's theories, then the area of endeavour is not science.

Although this is not the only view of what science is about, it is the one which predominates in modern psychology, with psychologists setting up theories, making predictions and testing them under specified conditions. Doubts have been expressed as to whether scientists do actually go about trying to disprove their theories—rather, they often seem quite keen on supporting them! But it may be true in a general sense that science progresses by the refutation process, even if one's theories are more likely to be challenged by others than by oneself.

There is, then, a fair degree of consensus that science, including psychological science, is about constructing and testing theories on the basis of systematically collected evidence. However, psychology has a problem which distinguishes it from the physical sciences, and that is its reflexive nature: people are the investigators, but people are also the subject matter. A lens isn't going to ask questions of an investigator; a chemical substance doesn't wonder what the purpose of an experiment is, but human subjects do, and psychologists must always endeavour to be aware of how this might affect the outcome or interpretation of a study.

It has been suggested that each of us is our own 'scientist', making hypotheses and predictions about the world and modifying our theories in the light of experience (Kelly, 1955). This has been taken further, to suggest that each of us is our own psychologist. We do, indeed, all have our own ideas about what makes people tick, and this enables us to function socially. This may lead us to believe that psychology is just common sense. The problem is that each of us has rather different ideas based on our own unique situation, and science is about trying to establish general rules which are agreed by a large number of experts in the field. Most parents hold views about child development based on experience with their own children, but general theories can only be arrived at by studying large numbers of children, looking for patterns, and trying to ascertain how differences might be explained. A psychologist must therefore try and remove biases in scientific investigations, by choosing subject samples carefully, by the use of appropriate comparison (control) groups and by using objective methods of data collection and analysis, in order to arrive at explanations which are as unambiguous as possible.

Experiments and statistics

Scientists usually aim to explain phenomena in predictive, cause-and-effect terms—that is, to be able to say: 'If x happens, the result will be y'. This is, to a large degree, possible in the physical sciences. Optometrists can predict, given the power of a lens, at what distance from it a clear image will be achieved, and it is possible to express the phenomenon of refraction in precise mathematical terms. This knowledge was built up through optical experiments in which lens power was systematically varied and its relationship with the vergence of incident and emergent light established. Unfortunately, things are not so simple in psychological research, nor indeed in optometric research when one is concerned not just with lenses but with a visual system which is part of a human being. Both ethical and practical reasons stand in the way of pure experimental design. If one wants to discover the psychological effects of visual loss, for example, one simply cannot take a group of people, blind them, and later compare them with a group of similar people not so treated.

Even in circumstances where experimental approaches are ethically acceptable as, for example, in many laboratory experiments on perception, memory and so on, questions of applicability to real life arise. One often has to be content, therefore, with manipulating conditions within the real world, utilizing what is called a quasi-experimental design—as many factors as possible are controlled, but there remains a greater degree of uncertainty with regard to cause and effect: y may follow from x because of the influence of some other related, unknown variable. In such a situation, one can conclude that x and y are correlated, that is, are systematically associated with one another, but not that one causes the other.

Even when an apparent effect is found in a study, such as when two groups of differently treated subjects differ on some measure, the question remains: Is this a real effect, or has it occurred by chance? This possibility must be considered because there are always unknown factors which could conceivably conspire to produce a certain misleading result once in a while. Psychologists make great use of statistical analysis, originally developed within the context of agriculture, to deal with this point. Optometrists involved in research increasingly do so too, but training in statistical methods does not form a major part of their education.

Statistics is a branch of mathematics concerned with the likelihood, or probability, of an event occurring by chance. If an experimenter applies treatment x to a single subject, and the outcome is y, it cannot be determined whether this was truly the result of the manipulation or due to some other, unknown variable—a chance happening. If the same treatment x resulted in y in 10 out of 10 subjects, one would be more confident that the effect was real. If it happened in 100 out of 100 subjects, one would be even more confident. But what if the predicted result occurred in only 90, or 80 subjects? Have you then a genuine effect or not? Statistics make it possible to calculate the probability of a result happening by chance (that is, to work out the level of confidence that any apparent effect is genuine), taking into account the particular experimental design and number of subjects in the study. By convention, the lowest level of acceptable statistical significance is a likelihood of that outcome occurring purely by chance on 1 out of 20 occasions (a probability of 0.05); however, a 1 in 100 chance (a probability of 0.01) is more acceptable. Confidence in the outcome is further increased if the study is replicated with similar results. Thus one form of bias in studies, using too small a sample, can be reduced by utilizing large numbers of experimental subjects and applying appropriate statistical techniques.

However, practical reasons may dictate that this is not possible. It may be too costly to use large numbers; to use a simple example, the more people sampled by a postal questionnaire, the more materials and postage will be needed, the more data will need to be analysed, necessitating more person-hours and computer time. Sometimes large studies are impossible because the phenomenon under study is a rare one, such as is the case with certain types of brain damage—for example, relatively few brain injuries lead to prosopagnosia, an inability to recognize faces (perhaps even one's own in a mirror) despite an otherwise intact visual system (Ellis, 1989). In such circumstances observations of small numbers and even single cases may be necessary. Standard statistical techniques are not applicable in such cases, but new methods are being developed which help the experimenter to maintain a degree of control, and prevent such studies from consisting simply of the subjective impressions of the investigator. Such methods, which rely on using an individual as his or her own control, rather than making comparisons between groups, are gaining increasing respectability (Barlow and Hersen, 1984).

Psychology and other sciences

Some psychologists argue that their discipline relies too much on experimental method as derived from the physical sciences, and favour the use of not only single-case designs, but of the systematic gathering of descriptive, qualitative information. Such systematic collection of evidence could perhaps be regarded as the bottom line in deciding whether an endeavour is scientific. This view would entail the rejection of Popper's definition of science, and hark back to the methods utilized in the early days of the physical sciences. It is perhaps appropriate that this level of enquiry should still be legitimate in psychology, which is often described as a 'young science': that is, it does not have any single paradigm within which all psychologists operate. Some refer to the 'psychological sciences' in the plural, and this is perhaps appropriate given the wide range of approaches to understanding human behaviour and experience already noted. While the predominant view is that this should mean the setting up and testing of hypotheses through controlled experiments, we have seen that this is not always feasible. The discipline therefore progresses by investigators approaching from a variety of angles in order each to contribute a little piece towards the construction of the overall puzzle.

The foregoing discussion makes it clear that psychologists have put an enormous amount of thought and effort into the methodology of their discipline, and this may stem from a recognition—perhaps only implicit—of the reflexive nature of the subject. Psychologists must endeavour to use objective methods to remove their own biases in observation and interpretation, to be aware of biases which may be introduced by the subject's perception of the investigation, and to take account of any limitations which the circumstances of data collection place upon inferences that can be drawn. Reflexivity also means that psychology must work harder than other sciences to get its findings accepted. Not many of us hold common-sense views about particle physics or biochemistry, but we do have our own ideas about the psychological functioning of ourselves and others, and so may need a lot of convincing about counterintuitive results.

However, the fact that psychology has had to do a great deal of soul-searching and indulge in self-criticism of its methodology should not mislead us into thinking that psychology is the only science with such problems. For example, observer bias—the tendency to see what one hopes or expects—is common to all sciences, and is something of which all scientists (and, indeed, clinicians) should beware. Few would question the scientific status of astronomy, yet it has been pointed out (Legge, 1981) that questions of control and cause and effect are even more problematical here than in psychology, since actual experiments are impossible—you cannot shift planets about to see what happens! Again, those working in other fields may have to deal with rare or uncontrollable phenomena: how many volcanic eruptions can a geologist hope to sample in a lifetime, and what controlled experiments can a meteorologist carry out on a tornado? Just like psychologists, these scientists must rely on small-scale experimentation and modelling to supplement real-life observations. The methodological stringency and self-awareness apparent in psychology are indicative not of the weakness, but of the strength of the discipline as a science.

Psychology and optometry

Psychologists have, of course, contributed a great deal to our understanding of vision. Some are engaged in research alongside optometrists, and members of the two professions make contact at interdisciplinary conferences and through the pages of journals devoted to vision. The term 'psycho-optometry' has been coined to cover the field of research and practice at the interface of psychology and optometry (Terry, 1989). So far, though, this term has been used mainly to refer to a small body of research on the psychological correlates of refractive corrections (for example, on how spectacle wearers are perceived by others). The majority of psychologists involved in optometry specialize in laboratory studies of visual processes, and are not generally involved with clinical practice. In particular, they do not appear to have been drawn into the movement of health psychology, which has much to offer optometry.

Although as yet few psychologists appreciate the direct contribution that their discipline could make to vision care, some practitioners are certainly aware of the importance of psychological factors within a clinical context. Those who have put pen to paper on the subject appear to have drawn upon a mixture of experience, common sense and psychological writings, although a lack of thorough documentation of sources often makes it difficult to determine from which particular fount of wisdom an individual pearl has been extracted. Practitioners who have acknowledged the importance of psychological aspects of their work have included the American ophthalmologists Milder and Rubin, whose book *The Fine Art of Prescribing Glasses Without Making a Spectacle of Yourself* (1978) was deemed best medical book of the year by the American Medical Writers' Association in 1979. It includes chapters entitled 'The psychodynamics of spectacle-wearing' and 'The dissatisfied refraction patient'. While I would take issue with the psychoanalytic flavour apparent at times in their book, credit is due to them and to Humphriss (1984), working in South Africa, for recognizing the importance of the simple fact that vision testing is carried out not on machines, but on people. A person's eyes are an integral part of the whole person, and cannot be considered in isolation.

However, Milder and Rubin were aware of the opposition that their views were likely to meet among some practitioners, who might fear that the intention was to turn them into amateur psychologists or psychiatrists. Similarly, Humphriss reported that some optometrists and ophthalmologists claim that refraction is a 'fully scientific' process which cannot be informed by psychology, which they regard as not properly scientific.

This misconception about the scientific status of the discipline has already been discussed, and the next chapter should make it clear that, quite contrary to the views of some refractionists as unearthed by Humphriss, refraction cannot possibly be carried out in a fully scientific manner without an understanding of the underlying psychological processes. As for the creation of amateur psychologists and psychiatrists out of optometrists, if by this it is meant that they should be aware of the importance of underlying psychological processes to the successful practice of their own profession, so be it: eyes cannot be divorced from the person.

The explosion of interest in health psychology in recent years has already been alluded to, and it has brought in its wake a growing recognition of the relevance of the discipline to a whole range of health care professions. Psychology is increasingly being incorporated into their training courses, and there has been a rash of textbooks aimed at those in various fields, including medicine, nursing, health visiting, physiotherapy, speech therapy and dentistry. Only one other book to date has been directed at optometric practice, and that is Humphriss's *Refraction Science and Psychology* (1984). Although it was written before the wealth of recent research within health psychology became available, and some aspects of the book are quite culture-specific, it does contain much useful information about aspects of clinical practice, particularly with regard to testing procedures. However, some of the research quoted remains unpublished, and is therefore unavailable for the critical scrutiny which is an essential part of the scientific process. Nevertheless, it appears to be the case that some of Humphriss' work is unique, and therefore certainly of interest, and the findings are at least suggestive. Some will be referred to in the course of this book on certain topics where there is no published research available; however, in the light of the foregoing discussion about scientific enquiry, it would clearly be desirable for these studies to be replicated and published.

Although some vision care practitioners are reported to be sceptical about the relevance of psychology to their profession, a glance through the popular optometry journals reveals a great deal of interest in psychological issues. Topics raised include the following: patient compliance (especially in relation to contact lens use); the patient–practitioner relationship; patient anxiety; the problems of missed appointments; the needs of special patient groups such as children with dyslexia, elderly people, those with intellectual impairments and those with hearing difficulties. Such articles frequently appear to be based on the anecdotes of practising optometrists rather than scientific investigations. Undoubtedly, valuable insights can be gained from examining the experiences of those working in practice, especially as it appears to be the case that little systematic research has been carried out on vision care. This book gathers together the small amount of research on optometric practice that does exist, together with relevant knowledge gained in related fields to augment the wisdom gained from clinical experience. How far such general lessons will need modifying within the context of optometry remains open to investigation. For example, much of the research on patient–practitioner relationships has been carried out in the field of medicine. It is not known how the relationship is affected when the patient is also a potential customer or client, as in pharmacy or optometry.

Despite the existence of such questions, as yet unanswered by empirical research, there are undoubtedly general issues of as much interest to vision care as to other health-related professions. One crucial factor they have in common is that they are face-to-face professions. Whereas many workers, such as motor mechanics, writers and pathologists, can carry out the greater part of their work alone, the optometrist's professional skills are utilized within an inherently interpersonal context. It is perhaps surprising, then, that the ability to communicate effectively with patients is not yet considered a vital part of training, and left almost entirely to chance. Undoubtedly, some individuals are naturally more socially skilled than others, and teachers of optometry will be able to think of certain academically and technically brilliant students whom they suspect will make less successful clinicians than those more mediocre students who have a 'good way with patients'. It is possible to develop good communication skills, and this is already part of the curriculum in the training of many other professional groups, through lectures, role-play and real-life exercises. No textbook on the issue is geared specifically towards vision care, and it is hoped that this book will offer some guidelines and act as a stimulus for the teaching not only of communication skills but of psychology in general on optometry courses, as well as being useful for individual students and practising optometrists wishing to enhance their clinical skills.

One way of structuring books on psychology aimed at other professional groups is to divide the subject matter in terms of traditional psychological topics, such as personality, intelligence, learning and memory. The present book approaches the material from the other end—the clinical situation—and examines topics which are of direct relevance. For example, it is probably not particularly helpful, in approaching a patient, to be armed with knowledge about personality and intelligence, since the optometrist will not be able to measure these, and it is not altogether clear what one should do with them if one could. Rather, the problem is one of trying to communicate effectively with the individual, of finding out what the patient already knows and expects, and of trying to get one's own viewpoint and advice across in a way that the patient is most likely to understand and remember. This involves insight into communication processes in general, together with a background understanding of the likely needs of particular patient groups—all this being aimed at helping the practitioner to understand 'where the patient is at' and where he or she wishes to go. As well as looking at communication and the needs of special groups, another important topic covered is that of the testing situation itself, which involves the patient in the psychological process of making subjective judgements about visual stimuli.

Although this book has been written with optometric practice in mind, those involved in vision care in other professional capacities will hopefully also find much to interest them. Chapter 8 on visual loss should be of particular interest to ophthalmologists and ophthalmic nurses, for example, while orthoptists are increasingly being asked to work with dyslexic children and those experiencing visual problems as a result of brain injury. All such professionals will find the chapters on patient–practitioner communication and dealing with special patient groups of relevance.

The value system underlying this consideration of the needs of special patients is the wish to see the potential of all such individuals fulfilled. Thorough visual assessment should be a vital step in rehabilitation and educational programmes, so that impaired vision can be enhanced if possible, and so that carers (and, as far as possible, the patients themselves) can structure their visual world in the most helpful way possible. Yet people such as those with intellectual impairment or multiple disabilities are frequently dismissed as too hard to test or even not worth testing.

However, patterns of health care are changing in some parts of the world, including the UK, Canada and the USA, and these changes may lead more optometrists to involve themselves in specialist aspects of vision care. Miller (1989) has discussed a range of changes which are taking place, including an increasing number of elderly in the population and the greater use of expensive, high-technology equipment, as well as political changes relating to the organization and financing of health care services. He has pointed out that under such pressures those practices that survive 'will probably be heavily oriented towards the provision of one or more areas of specialized optometric care'. Those who are looking to specialize, if only partially, in particular client groups, might consider patients with special needs. It would be possible, for instance, to set aside a certain number of hours a week to run a clinic for infants or low vision patients, or arrange to visit a nearby hospital or day centre catering for people who have had strokes or those with multiple impairments. It is hoped that this volume offers a deeper understanding of the needs of such patient groups and that this, together with a consideration of some specific assessment techniques, will make the taking on of such patients seem a more approachable task. I and my colleagues from the Visual Assessment Unit and Low Vision Clinic within University of Wales College of Cardiff's Department of Optometry can vouch for the interest, variety and reward that come from working with patients with special needs.

References

Barlow D.H., Hersen M. (1984). *Single Case Experimental Designs: Strategies for Studying Behaviour* Change 2nd ed. New York: Pergamon.

Ellis H.D. (1989). Past and recent studies of prosopagnosia. In *Developments in Clinical and Experimental Neuropsychology* (Crawford J.R., Parker., D.M. eds). New York: Plenum.

Farrell B.A. (1963). Psychoanalysis — II. The method. *New Society*, **39**, 12–14.

Humphriss D. (1984). *Refraction Science and Psychology*. Cape Town: Juta.

Johnston M. (1990). Behaviour, health and disease. In: *Psychology and Health Promotion* (Shute R.H., Penny G.N., eds). Cardiff: British Psychological Society, Welsh Branch.

Kelly G. (1955). *A Theory of Personality: The Psychology of Personal Constructs*. New York: Norton.

Legerton J. (1989). How personable are you? *Rev. Optom.*, March 29–31.

Legge D. (1981). Scientific methodology. In *Psychology for Physiotherapists*. (Dunkin E.N., ed.). London: Macmillan Press British Psychological Society.

Mace C.A., ed. (1957). *British Philosophy in the Mid-Century*. London: Allen and Unwin, p. 159.

Milder B., Rubin M.L. (1978). *The Fine Art of Prescribing Glasses Without Making a Spectacle of Yourself*. Gainesville, FL: Triad Scientific Publications.

Miller S.C. (1989). Impact of health care trends on the practice of optometry. *Optom. Vision Sci.*, **66**, 698–704.

Roberts E. (1988). The psychology of fitting RGP lenses. *Rev. Optom.*, April, 25–6.

Shute R.H. (1986). 'It's worse than going to the dentist' — identifying and dealing with anxiety in optical practice. *Optical Manage.*, October 10–12.

Shute R., Penny G.N. (1989). Health-related counselling: control, coping and communication. *Counselling Psychol. Q.*, **2**, 245–7.

Terry R.L. (1989). Eyeglasses and gender stereotypes. *Optom. Vision Sci.*, **66**, 694–7.

Wilkinson S.R. (1988). *The Child's World of Illness: The Development of Health and Illness Behaviour*. Cambridge: Cambridge University Press.

Chapter 2

Perception and procedures in vision testing

Introduction

This chapter and the next examine two categories of psychological processes which are inherent aspects of vision care: the perceptual and the social. Although traditionally these topics are distinct areas of enquiry and highlighted here in separate chapters, they are, in reality, closely linked. For example, the way someone perceives or responds to a visual stimulus can be affected by social circumstances, such as what another person has led him or her to expect. Conversely, the social processes involved in making judgements about other people are sometimes referred to as 'person perception'. Visual perceptual and social factors interweave during the course of an optometric consultation and are normally taken completely for granted. These hidden processes are important, however, as they help to determine how a patient responds to optometric testing.

Visual perception is considered first since traditionally trained optometrists are likely to feel more at home with this subject than with social psychology. Much of what goes on in an optometric consultation is concerned with how patients perceive the visual stimuli with which they are presented or, to be more accurate, since their perceptions are not directly accessible to the optometrist, with how they respond to those perceptions. In this chapter, discussion centres on the nature of visual perception and on some factors which can influence responses to the kinds of visual tasks typically presented during optometric testing.

What is perception?

Specifying the nature of visual perception is a thorny problem on which there is not universal agreement (Katz, 1982; McArthur, 1982). While vision is commonly referred to as one of the senses, sensory and perceptual systems need to be distinguished from one another, according to Gibson (1966). He proposed that the essential difference is that sensory systems are concerned with energy (light energy, or photons, in the case of vision), while perception is concerned with information. The difference can be illustrated by considering two simple optometric tests. When an optometrist uses a pen torch to test pupillary responses a sensory system is being examined—the tester is checking that the pupil will respond appropriately to the amount of light energy impinging on the eye. However, when a patient is asked to name a letter on a Snellen chart, information from the pattern of light, indicating the shape of the letter, is needed in order to identify it.

Gibson's approach appears to be well accepted in this respect. However, another aspect of his theory is more controversial. He maintained that all perception occurs *directly*, through the extraction of information carried in the light reaching the perceiver's eyes. Taking such a view, when a patient sees a letter on a Snellen chart, all the information necessary for identifying it is contained in the pattern of reflected light.

While this view that perception is direct is arguably possible when considering the perceptual processes of a creature such as a fly, it is difficult to support in the case of higher organisms, especially people (Fodor and Pylyshyn, 1981). Bruce and Green (1989) have argued convincingly that almost everything we perceive visually involves the processing of information from sources other than the incoming light: that is, most visual perception is *indirect*. It necessitates some element of higher, cognitive, processing, which involves internal representations of the world. They have drawn attention to the difference between seeing and seeing *as*. Most human activity takes place within a cultural environment, and people see objects and events *as* what they are in terms of a culturally determined representation of the world, and processes such as memory and expectation play a part in determining perceptions.

A good example is the 'hollow face' illusion (Gregory, 1973). If the inside surface of a hollow facemask is viewed from a few feet away, it appears to be a normal face, with the nose pointing towards the observer. The information contained in the light reflected from the mask is over-ridden by other information—the viewer's knowledge that faces stick out and are not hollow. That perception depends on experience of the visual world is also indicated by the problems faced by people whose sight is restored following the removal of childhood cataracts. They have great difficulty in making sense of the visual world: they can *see*, but not see *as*. At first, they can only recognize an object after touching it; the visual information must be integrated with their existing knowledge of the world to create new representations which incorporate visual as well as tactile information.

Even in cases where it can be argued that perception occurs without any intervening cognitive processes such as memory, judgement, expectations and so on, theorists such as Marr (1982) have argued that perception is still not direct. He argued that automatic 'computations' by the visual system must intervene so that the information in the observed pattern of light can be used. An example is the process by which the edges of objects and surfaces are detected by means of computations based on intensity changes in the pattern of light reaching the eye.

There is, then, a strong body of opinion against the Gibsonian view that perception occurs directly. Processing visual information seems to involve, at a minimum, the performance of computations and, in human beings, will usually involve higher cognitive processes also.

That perception is no simple matter was apparent from the earliest psychophysical studies, devised in order to catalogue the abilities of the senses to detect differences in stimulus energy. One of the foremost early workers in this area was Fechner. Much of his most influential work was carried out in the 1830s, and he helped to establish the science of experimental psychology. It was Fechner who coined the term 'psychophysics' and it is ironic, given the subject matter of this book, that he damaged his eyes by gazing at the sun through coloured glasses while carrying out research on after-sensations (Thomson, 1968). In visual psychophysics, a mea-sured change is made in some aspect of the physical energy impinging upon the visual system in order to find out if this change makes any difference to what the observer perceives. Both absolute thresholds and discrimination thresholds (just noticeable differ-ences, or JNDs) have been the object of study (Hochberg, 1964). Both types are of interest in optometric testing. For example, a contrast sensitivity test measures an absolute threshold, while discrimination thresholds are involved during refraction when a patient is asked which of two lenses makes the target appear clearer.

It has long been recognized that such perceptual thresholds are not simple, fixed values. When an individual is asked to make judgements about whether two very similar stimuli are identical or not, fluctuations in response will occur, so that the two stimuli may be judged as the same on one occasion and different on another. It was a television engineer (Rose, 1942) who first suggested that visual discrimination might be affected by 'noise' in the visual system. This view was later developed further, so that perception came to be seen as an active process, with the brain deciding whether a change in neural impulse rate is a chance happening, or a significant event to be accepted as a real signal (Gregory, 1966).

The level above which a change is to be accepted as a signal is not fixed, and is affected by variations in motivation and expectation. This was established in the mid 20th century through experiments which varied the conditions under which identical stimuli were viewed. If, for example, people were shown blurred pictures of food which were gradually brought into focus, hungry subjects would identify the pictures sooner than those who were not hungry (McClelland and Atkinson, 1948). Another example is afforded by the well known ambiguous drawing which can be perceived as either a young woman or an old woman: it will be differently perceived by a naive observer depending on whether a slightly different drawing shown beforehand more closely resembles the old or the young woman (Leeper, 1935). Even something as apparently simple as judging the size of a circular poker chip can be affected by prior experience: if the chips are given value by allowing the subjects to trade them for rewards, they are judged as bigger (Lambert et al., 1949).

Influences on perceptual responding in vision testing

How far such considerations are relevant within the context of vision care will depend on the degree to which vision tests involve cognition, rather than just computational processes. Although optometric testing is aimed at assessing only basic visual functions rather than more complex perceptual abilities, we have already seen that even something as apparently simple as establishing a visual threshold can involve cognition. There seems no reason to suppose that the kinds of influence on visual judgements demonstrated in the laboratory will be any less operative in a clinical situation. A patient, like a subject in a psychophysical experiment, is required to make judgements about visual stimuli, frequently at threshold. For example, the duochrome test to assess the best vision sphere is aimed at establishing a discrimination threshold, while acuity and contrast sensitivity tests determine absolute thresholds.

Within an optometric context, the distinction between perception with and without cognitive involvement can be illustrated by considering visual acuity. This can be measured via several different routes, depending on whether a detection, resolution or recognition task is used, and on the nature of response required. It is perhaps possible to consider detection and resolution tests as involving direct perception in the Gibsonian sense or, at any rate, as involving computational rather than cognitive processes. For example, when acuity is measured by means of the Catford drum all that is required is the automatic detection of a moving target (Catford and Oliver, 1971), a process which normally occurs without any cognitive involvement. Similarly, when acuity is measured in a young baby using acuity cards (see Chapter 5), the infant simply looks towards the grating in preference to a blank target if he or she can resolve the pattern. In both these cases the patient is, arguably, responding purely to the information contained in the light reflected from the test materials.

However, such examples of vision tests which involve only direct perception or computational processes are rare. Acuity, to continue with our example, is more commonly measured using recognition tasks, which draw on sources of information other than the pattern of incoming light: for example, memory and naming processes are required to identify letters on a Snellen chart. Even otherwise direct tests can become indirect if the procedure is changed, as when acuity cards are used with a toddler who is asked to point to the stripes: the child must draw upon his or her understanding of the words. Similarly, if an infant is taught the task by being reinforced (rewarded) for looking towards the grating, then perception will again be indirect, as learning is involved. So, just as it has been argued that most perceptual tasks in everyday life involve cognitive processes, it seems that the same is true of most clinical vision tests, which are therefore likely to be influenced by such factors as the patient's motivation and expectation.

At this point, it is important to recall the perhaps obvious fact that the optometrist does not have direct access to the patient's perceptions, as these are filtered through the mechanisms necessary for the patient to respond to the test; for example, a patient who cannot speak cannot name a letter on a Snellen chart even if he or she can recognize it. Furthermore, extraneous influences may affect not just the perception itself, but the decision on how to respond— for example, whether or not to hazard a guess about a stimulus one is uncertain about.

Such influences on the eventual response to a visual stimulus are normally taken for granted in vision testing. The average patient will be an adult who can, and is willing to, read a Snellen chart, for example, and it is for just such patients that most tests have been devised. However, when children or special patients are being tested standard approaches, tests and procedures may be inappropriate: consideration must be given to whether the patient has the necessary cognitive (and physical) skills which the test presupposes. As Lindstedt (1986) has discussed, the skills that may be presupposed by standard tests include attentiveness, memory, ability to generalize, understanding of concepts such as similar/different and ability to communicate by spoken language or signs. Some or all of these abilities may be impaired in certain patients such as the very young, those with intellectual impairments and those who have suffered strokes.

While certain factors which influence responding are brought into sharp focus with certain patients, such as those with communication or memory problems, subtle influences on test responses that are operative with all patients must not be overlooked. Humphriss (1984) is one of the few previous workers to draw attention to this. Although much of his supporting evidence is not published in detail, and would certainly benefit from replication, it remains the only comprehensive effort to examine influences on responding to optometric tests. The factors discussed by Humphriss include individual differences in perception, the instructions given by the tester, the procedures utilized and the test design itself. Each of these will now be considered in more detail.

Individual differences in perception

Humphriss, quite rightly, was concerned about individual differences between patients. However, my own view is that his approach, in terms of different personality types, although intrinsically interesting, is not particularly helpful clinically. While various personality classifications have been drawn up (and may indeed be related to different ways of seeing the world, as Humphriss's evidence and that of other researchers suggests) it is only possible to classify an individual as introverted or whatever by means of specially devised tests; this is not something which the optometrist will, or should, be doing. At best, he or she might hazard some kind of guess about a patient's personality, but this would not lead to any particularly obvious course of action, and could well represent a stereotyping process which, it is argued in the next chapter, should be avoided. It must nevertheless be recognized that patients do differ in the ways they approach the consultation, both in a general sense and in terms of the sight testing itself. The proposal here is that these differences are best dealt with in three ways.

Firstly, the optometrist should be responsive to the likely needs of different kinds of patient, such as the elderly, children or those suffering visual loss; other chapters in this book are aimed at giving background information on the likely needs of such groups. However, this only takes us to the point of regarding people as members of groups, and the argument about avoiding stereotyping still applies. Although general, factually derived guidelines are helpful for getting the optometrist into the right ballpark, as it were, the needs of all children or all people with brain injuries are not the same.

This brings us to the second way of dealing with individual differences. The optometrist must respond sensitively to events as they unfold during the course of the consultation. This is discussed in Chapters 4 and 5, which suggest specific ways of dealing with individual patients' concerns and with the problem of the patient who is not forthcoming in discussing case history, special worries and so forth.

Thirdly, it must be acknowledged that patients will vary in the ways in which they respond to the sight testing itself; for example, a more cautious responder will appear to have a more restricted visual field. Although my view is that Humphriss's approach, in terms of personality types, is inappropriate, his solution for dealing with possible individual biases in responding seems perfectly sound: to use test procedures which preclude the various types of response biases which may exist. This will be discussed further below.

Instructions

With few exceptions, such as the tests mentioned earlier which seem to involve only direct perception or computational vision, most aspects of vision testing necessitate some kind of instructions being given to the patient. Sometimes the co-operation required is minimal, such as when carrying out ophthalmoscopy, objective refraction or measuring intraocular pressure, but even these procedures become difficult if the patient cannot respond to instructions to turn his or her eyes in the appropriate direction. More often, the active co-operation of patients is needed in indicating their perception of presented targets. We have already seen that perception itself can be influenced by expectations which have been set up by someone else, and this suggests that the optometrist needs to exercise care in giving instructions so as not to bias the way the patient sees the presented stimuli. In addition, care must be taken so that the patient is clear about the type of response that is acceptable, and to avoid creating anxiety.

As discussed by Humphriss, many patients will be anxious to some degree about vision testing. The very terms often used to describe the situation, such as 'sight test' and 'eye examination' may conjure up anxiety-arousing associations such as school examinations and driving tests, and the use of alternatives such as 'vision care' and 'eye care' by a practice may help to set an alternative ethos. Similarly, the use of the word 'patient' may be associated with worrying medical situations (the use of this word may be undesirable for other reasons too, as will be discussed later in the book). It was noted earlier that patients are often required to make judgements in order to establish thresholds, so the tasks are inherently difficult as threshold is reached. Anxiety about performance is therefore likely, and the patient may be concerned about whether to guess or about giving wrong answers. Anxiety can influence visual perception or, at least, the response to it, as shown by an experiment in which subjects were found to need more time to identify nonsense syllables which had previously been associated with electric shock (McGinnies, 1949). According to Humphriss, an anxious patient is more difficult to test satisfactorily, being inclined to make more errors.

One purpose of the instructions given to the patient should therefore be to reduce anxiety. Sometimes it may be more of an explanation than an instruction which is required, so that the patient knows what to expect and is not made more anxious by unexpected events. Otherwise, instructions should be aimed at reducing any feeling that the patient is somehow on trial. Other specific sources of anxiety, apart from this natural performance anxiety, should be detected and dealt with during the taking of the case history or at any stage during testing if the patient suddenly opens up (see Chapters 4 and 5).

Humphriss has suggested that, before refraction, patients are given instructions aimed at reducing anxiety and ensuring that they understand what is required. He suggests that patients should be told, firstly, not to worry about mistakes, nor to change their answers, as each will be cross-checked; secondly, they should be told not to worry about very small differences in choosing between the clarity of two lenses, but to judge them as the same; thirdly, patients should be told that all questions will be asked twice, and they should give their answer first time if they are sure of it, or after the second if not. Humphriss presents these instructions in the form of a kind of standard speech over 100 words long, comprising three sections, each with a conditional component (of the 'if. . . then. . .' type); he seems to be suggesting that this should be delivered before refraction. As discussed in a later chapter, patients often find it difficult to take in detailed instructions or explanations, particularly if the language is complex, therefore it seems likely that giving all these details at one hearing could be counterproductive and even create more anxiety.

It is preferable, therefore, to make the various points at appropriate moments during the test procedures, once the patient has got the feel of what is going on. At the outset, some kind of general comment such as the following may be appropriate: 'I'll explain what I'd like you to do as we go along. If you think you've given a wrong answer don't worry about it—I expect that to happen, and my procedures are designed to handle it'. Actions may, in any case, speak louder than words, and Humphriss' suggestion that a trial run with easy targets should be used to augment explanations is an excellent one.

Communicating instructions will be facilitated if the optometrist uses language understood by the patient. This is discussed in more detail in Chapter 4, but we can note here an example given by Humphriss in relation to testing a young child's stereoacuity with the Frisby test. While we may see the task as looking for a circle in a square, a young child is more likely to see it as looking for the ball in the box—where possible, the child's own descriptions should be ascertained beforehand and used.

Action, rather than a verbal explanation, may be vital with patients who have difficulty in dealing with spoken instructions. This might include some young children, some patients with an intellectual impairment and some who have certain types of language problem as a result of brain damage. This will be discussed further in the relevant chapters, but at the moment the general point can be made that a technique known as operant conditioning can be very useful in such instances.

This technique comes from the behaviourist tradition of psychology. The idea is that the patient receives a reward for giving an appropriate response, a process known as reinforcement. Training should utilize targets which the patient is expected to see easily. Depending on the particular patient, simple social reinforcement may be sufficient, such as saying 'good', 'well done', 'that's right', and smiling and nodding. Some babies are delighted to receive applause for an appropriate response, and toys and glove puppets which appear when a correct response is given can be invaluable for getting the message across. In exceptional cases, and with a carer's permission (or even at their suggestion), it may be necessary to resort to food or drink. If so, this should be meted out in small quantities contingent on correct responding, for example, one potato crisp per correct response: the patient who is handed the whole packet has little motivation to attend to sight testing! Protecting costly equipment such as acuity cards from sticky fingers is also advisable; presenting them behind perspex sheets is suitable, provided care is taken to avoid reflections from room lights (Leat, personal communication).

Procedures

One aspect of procedure that needs to be considered is which tests should be carried out, and in what order. Clearly, there will be certain tests which the optometrist will aim to carry out with all patients, while case history may suggest the necessity for other tests with certain patients. However, some tests may interfere with performance on later tests, as when patients learn a Snellen chart through repeat testing (alternative charts should be available, and stored out of sight). Some patients may have a limited attention span: perhaps they fatigue easily or are on certain medication; infants between 1 and 2 years may be particularly upset by certain procedures or prolonged testing (Shute et al., 1990). If extensive testing is necessary a return visit to complete it might be indicated.

Otherwise, the practitioner needs to make a decision about what seem the most important tests to carry out and whether these should therefore be attempted first. For example, as Humphriss has discussed, there is much to be said for leaving ophthalmoscopy until last, as it is not particularly pleasant and may therefore create anxiety as well as an afterimage, both of which may interfere with later vision tests. However, an ophthalmologist may feel it appropriate to do this first because the primary interest is the detection of pathology, which is far more prevalent in the ophthalmologist's patient population than the optometrist's.

Once a decision about order of testing has been made, and some kind of initial instructions about a particular test have been given, testing can begin. The optometrist should have an overall plan as to what procedure to follow, but will be adapting it according to how the patient responds. We can think in terms of the general way in which the tester handles the patient, and of specific procedures aimed at reducing biased responding.

Firstly, the tester must continue to be aware of the possibility of anxiety, especially as thresholds are approached and the patient becomes unsure. As long ago as 1955 it was demonstrated that how people respond to blurred images can be affected by how the examiner treats them. Subjects were shown blurred pictures which gradually increased in clarity; those who were reproached for their inability to identify the early, very blurred, images began guessing earlier, but made more errors, in comparison with subjects who were reassured about their performance (Smock, 1955). The implication is that reassuring patients is important, and this can be done by such comments as 'good', 'well done' or 'that's fine' even when, or especially when, they have reached their limit. Certainly, it seems likely that irritation with a patient who is proving difficult to test will make things worse.

The question of response bias can be tackled by appropriate procedures. Humphriss regarded one type of bias, perseveration, as of particular importance for binocular refraction. This occurs when, for example, a person perceives an ambiguous figure in one way, and is unable to see the alternative. Humphriss demonstrated that stereoscopically normal subjects fell into two clear groups with respect to their ability to change their perception of a synoptophore slide from a monocular to a binocular percept, some taking considerably longer or failing to change percept altogether. Humphriss maintained that such individuals will be difficult to refract using the duochrome technique as they will keep giving the same answer. Similarly, when asked to make judgements about cross-cylinders, some patients always report that the second position is better (Leat, personal communication). Humphriss's solution to this, for both the duochrome technique and cross-cylinders, is to use bracketing. The general idea is that, instead of creeping gradually closer to the presumed target, the tester establishes a bracket within which the end-point lies; the size of the bracket is then reduced until the patient cannot say which of two choices is better, and the middle of the bracket is taken as the correct answer. There seems no reason not to use this procedure for all patients, as the tester is not likely to know in advance whether or not a particular patient is a perseverator [the reader is referred to Humphriss (1984) for a more detailed discussion of bracketing].

Perseveration is one kind of response bias. Another, mentioned earlier, is whether a patient is characteristically cautious or not in responding. For example, a cautious responder may appear to have a reduced visual field in comparison with someone more willing to guess, but then the guesser is expected to make more false positive responses. This is conventionally dealt with by repeat testing, and taking the threshold as the point which is detected on 75% of occasions. Furthermore, as far as field testing is concerned, asymmetries may be more important than actual size, unless there are reasons for suspecting the presence of tunnel vision. Cautious responders may appear to have a lower acuity on a Snellen chart, therefore it is important to encourage patients to guess if their acuity is unexpectedly low. However, Humphriss suggests that this should not be done during the initial warm-up and that testing should cease as soon as the patient hesitates so as not to increase anxiety early on in testing.

Asking questions precisely is another important aspect of procedure. Again, it is the duochrome test in which the examiner may create problems through using a sloppy mode of questioning. The question is not, 'Which is clearer, the red or the green?' but 'Which circles appear clearer, those on the red or those on the green?'. In fact, there is a third alternative, that there is no difference, and this option should always be given in comparing lenses, otherwise many patients who cannot perceive any difference will be inhibited from saying so.

Hitherto, discussion has centred on the patient's perceptions, but we must not forget that the tester's perceptions also play a part, and the optometrist may make judgements influenced by what he or she expects to find. A good example of this is in testing an infant's acuity with acuity cards. If the tester knows in advance which side the target (a grating of known spatial frequency) is on, it is all too easy to wait for the baby to look that way and then accept that as the response! This can be avoided by giving the test blind—only checking on the correctness of the response after first making a decision as to where the baby was looking. In general, however, little appears to be known about the test–retest reliability of tester judgements made during optometric testing, and this is an area where research would certainly be worthwhile.

Biases in test materials

It is possible for test materials themselves to bias the kind of response an observer gives. Experimentally, this has been demonstrated by the finding that a reversed image of a letter of the alphabet requires a longer exposure before being correctly identified than the actual letter (Henle, 1942). A similar process has been suggested as being operative in the case of the Landolt C (Pointer, 1986). It has been shown that indecisive observers are more likely to guess that the break in the standard ring is to the right, but that this bias disappears using a more angular version of the target which is less reminiscent of the letter C.

Of course, a bias such as this is not really inherent in the test, but exists in the perceiver. The fact that we are willing to consider a bias as existing in the test itself is an indication that we are making culturally biased assumptions about what the test is likely to mean for most patients. Giving careful thought to the abilities needed for any particular test is a particularly useful exercise when it comes to deciding which tests and procedures are most appropriately used with which patients. Further consideration of this will be given in the chapters dealing with special patient groups.

Conclusions

Despite the problems which subjective tests involve, they have the advantage of permitting non-invasive assessments of visual function to be made, and cannot be entirely replaced by more objective tests; for example, measurement of intraocular pressure in glaucoma does not in itself indicate whether vision has been damaged. The range of available tests is being increased all the time: standard tests such as Snellen acuity charts are being joined by new tests to measure such functions as spatial and temporal contrast sensitivity, perimetric rod and cone sensitivity, colour vision and hyperacuity thresholds (Fitzke, 1988). It has been argued in this chapter that most such tests involve complex perceptual processes which can affect the ease and effectiveness of testing. Some ways of dealing with this, such as taking care with instructions given to patients and avoiding the creation of anxiety, have been suggested.

References

Bruce V., Green P. (1989). *Visual Perception: Physiology, Psychology and Ecology*. Hove: Lawrence Erlbaum.
Catford G.V., Oliver A. (1971). A method of visual acuity detection. In

Proceedings of Second International Orthoptic Congress. Amsterdam: Excerpta Medica, pp. 183–7.

Fitzke F.W. (1988). Clinical psychophysics. *Eye*, **2**, (suppl.), S 233–41.

Fodor J.A., Pylyshyn Z.W. (1981). How direct is visual perception? Some reflections on Gibson's 'Ecological Approach'. *Cognition*, **9**, 139–96.

Gibson J.J. (1966). *The Senses Considered as Perceptual Systems*. Boston: Houghton Mifflin.

Gregory R.L. (1966). *Eye and Brain*. London: Weidenfeld and Nicolson.

Gregory R. L. (1973). The confounded eye. In *Illusion in Nature and Art* (Gregory R.L., Gombrich E.H., Eds)., London: Duckworth.

Henle M. (1942). An experimental investigation of past experiences as a determinant of visual form perception. *J. Exp. Psychol.*, **30**, 1–22.

Hochberg J.E. (1964). *Perception*. Englewood Cliffs, NJ: Prentice-Hall.

Humphriss D. (1984). *Refraction Science and Psychology*. Cape Town: Juta.

Katz S. (1982). R.L. Gregory and others: the wrong picture of the picture theory of perception. *Perception*, **12**, 269–79.

Lambert W., Solomon R., Watson P. (1949). Reinforcement and extinction as factors in size estimation. *J. Exp. Psychol.*, **39**, 637–41.

Leeper R. (1935). A study of a neglected portion of the field of learning: the development of sensory organisation. *J. Gen. Psychol.*, **46**, 41–75.

Lindstedt E. (1986). Early vision assessment in visually handicapped children at the TRC, Sweden. *Br. J. Visual Impairment*, **IV**, 249–51.

Marr D. (1982). *Vision: A Computational Investigation into the Human Representation and Processing of Visual Information*. San Francisco: W.H. Freeman.

McArthur D.J. (1982). Computer vision and perceptual psychology. *Psychol. Bull.*, **92**, 283–309.

McClelland D., Atkinson J. (1948). The projective expression of needs. I. The effect of different intensities of the hunger drive on perception. *J. Psychol.*, **25**, 205–22.

McGinnies E. (1949). Emotionality and perceptual defense. *Psychol. Rev.*, **16**, 244–51.

Pointer J.S. (1986). Toward the elimination of guessing bias in Landolt acuity testing. *Am. J. Optom. Physiol. Opt.*, **63**, 813–18.

Rose A. (1942). The relative sensitivities of television pick-up tubes, photographic film and the human eye. *Proc. Inst. Radio Eng.*, **30**, 293.

Shute R., Candy R., Westall C., Woodhouse M.J. (1990). Success rates in testing monocular acuity and stereopsis in infants and young children. *Ophthalmic Physiol. Opt.*, **10**, 133–6.

Smock C.D. (1955). The influence of psychological stress on the tolerance of ambiguity. *J. Abnormal Social Psychol.*, **50**, 177.

Thomson R. (1968). *The Pelican History of Psychology*. Harmondsworth: Penguin.

Chapter 3

Social psychological aspects of vision care

Introduction

Although the previous chapter focused on perceptual processes in vision care, it also made it clear that it is almost impossible to consider these without simultaneously taking account of social factors, such as the instructions given by the optometrist to the patient. There are some wider social psychological issues also of relevance to optometric practice, and these are considered in this chapter and also the next, which deals specifically with communication.

Before a patient even walks through the door, the optometrist will have certain ideas about patients in a general sense and the role he or she as an optometrist expects to fulfil, *vis-à-vis* those patients. The social role of the practitioner (and the corresponding role of patient) is therefore an important aspect of vision care. Another is the fact that central to optometric practice, as to all face-to-face professions, is the need to meet and deal with members of the public, most of whom will be relative or complete strangers; the practitioner will begin to form an impression of each right from the first moment, and these initial perceptions help to set the tone of the consultation. Finally, when it comes to prescribing, considering the social significance of the eyes and visual correctives can give the optometrist insight into some concerns which patients may have with respect to the wearing of spectacles or contact lenses.

The Roles of Patient and Practitioner

Role Theory and Optometry

First, consideration needs to be given to the way in which the optometrist perceives patients in a general sense, as this will form the backdrop upon which interactions with individual patients are superimposed.

Social psychologists use the term 'role' to refer to the set of behaviours prescribed for or expected of a person occupying a certain position in the social structure (Robinson, 1972). Examples of roles are parent, citizen, daughter, husband and teacher. Individuals will occupy a number of roles simultaneously, their roles will change throughout life, and the demands of certain roles will change with societal changes. Some roles form complementary pairs, such as parent–child, husband–wife and teacher–pupil; patient and practitioner are another instance of roles which complement each other. Within any such role relationship, the people concerned may differ in status, that is to say, the higher status person is perceived as having the right to a degree of control over the other person's behaviour regardless of that person's wishes. Examples are parent–child relationships and doctor–patient relationships of the 'doctor knows best' type. Research has shown that general practitioners vary in their consultation styles, some being more authoritarian than others (Byrne and Long, 1976), and this is probably dependent at least in part on how the doctor sees his or her role. There is little evidence as to the origins of these role perceptions, but they are presumably influenced by personality differences and learning experiences in medical school and in later training (Weinman, 1987).

No research appears to have been carried out directly on how optometrists and their patients see their respective roles, although professional organizations may specify the role that practitioners are expected to fulfil. For example, the Canadian Association of Optometrists (1985) has published a role statement which lays down responsibilities in the eight areas of prevention, health education, health promotion, health maintenance, diagnosis, treatment and rehabilitation, counselling and consultation. Optometrists are presumably socialized into fulfilling such roles during the course of their training and through later contact with the profession through journals, conferences and so on.

They are probably also influenced in more subtle, covert ways. Bearing in mind that adopting a role involves assimilating the trappings that go with it, including styles of dress, the following university optometry department regulation is of interest:

> White jackets are compulsory for third-year students during clinic sessions and all hospital visits. Students are asked to dress respectably, and in particular, jeans should not be worn.

White jackets are rarely needed in optometry for the purposes of cleanliness, and the only practical purpose that appears to have been ascribed to them is the fact that they have pockets which are useful for such items as pens and PD rule (Humphriss, 1984). I suspect that their primary purpose is to place the student in the role of 'respectable professional'. White coats are strongly associated with doctors, so there may be the wish to cloak the profession with the high-status trappings of medicine. It is perhaps ironic, therefore, that recent years have seen a move away from the old authoritarian doctor–patient relationship towards the adoption of a more collaborative, egalitarian consultative style.

This change has been noted among the health-related professions in general, fostering a situation within which patients can accept a greater responsibility for their health and play a more active part in its promotion (Dickson, 1989). Gardner and McCormack (1990) have drawn attention to Peters's (1966) distinction between being *in* authority (on the basis of status) and being *an* authority (on the basis of expertise), and suggest that the health professional today should be the latter rather than the former.

Miller (1989) has noted that today's optometrists function as primary health care professionals whose services must be co-ordinated with those of other health care workers, and that they are not immune to the many forces and trends at work in the health care field: 'The same issues that affect the delivery of medical care will ultimately affect optometric care'. It seems reasonable to suppose, therefore, that those attending for vision care today will increasingly be expecting the roles of patient and optometrist to be complementary but egalitarian, and that optometrists will have to adjust their own perspective accordingly.

Indeed, it is questionable whether the term 'patient' should be retained at all, in view of the passive implications it has, and the term 'client', which does not have status implications, may be more appropriate. This may be particularly relevant in the case of those with special needs, such as low vision. Dodds (1988) has pointed out that such people may have received repeated messages from health care workers and others that they are helpless, and that this may stand in the way of their ability to manage their own lives effectively; the use of the word 'patient' may reinforce this helpless image. His reference to mobility training for the visually impaired has general applicability: he points out that it is the role of the trainer to *enable* rather than *disable* the client, and that this can only be achieved by an egalitarian, rather than an authoritarian, approach.

Despite this, I have nevertheless chosen to retain the term 'patient' in this book! This is because its primary purpose is to take the messages of psychology into vision care, and communicating messages is facilitated by adopting the language codes of the person receiving the message. It is my hope, though, that by the end of the book some readers will have been convinced enough by the general approach to conclude for themselves that the term 'client' is indeed more suitable for those who seek their professional services. This general approach can be summarised as a client-centred approach, which focuses on the individuality of each person seeking vision care.

The optometrist as counsellor

If the patient is to have a say in the consultation, it follows that the optometrist must avoid seeing vision care as something which is done *to* the patient *by* the practitioner. Research in various medical and paramedical settings has indicated that patients are not passive entities, even within the old authority-based patient–practitioner relationship: they bring with them certain expectations and beliefs which affect the progress of the consultation, and the practitioner ignores this to the detriment of patient care and satisfaction. This will be considered in detail in the following chapter, which places the onus on the professional to manage the dialogue with the patient in as productive a way as possible.

In becoming an authority rather than being in authority, the optometrist will find himself or herself acting in the role of counsellor. Not all health care practitioners will have thought of themselves as counsellors, but some aspects of counselling, such as giving information and advice to patients, are an inescapable part of the job. Good counselling also involves the skills of listening and attending. Heron (1986) has described six different types of verbal intervention which the counsellor may use at various times: prescriptive, informative, confronting, cathartic, catalytic and supportive.

Prescriptive interventions are those in which the practitioner advises a particular course of action; this type of intervention should not be overused, or the professional will slip back towards being in authority rather than an authority, appearing heavy-handed, dominating and patronizing. Informative interventions are related to practical issues, such as explaining to patients how to care for their contact lenses or use low vision aids. Confrontation challenges the patient to face a particular issue, but not in an aggressive way; it needs sensitive use and is discussed further in the following chapter. Cathartic interventions involve allowing the patient to express strong emotion, such as in the case of a tearful or angry patient who is trying to come to terms with visual loss. Catalytic interventions draw a patient out, encouraging discussion and finding out how much he or she knows about the situation at hand; this is achieved by appropriate questioning and body language, which are also discussed further in the next chapter. The final sort of intervention involves support, such as when the optometrist tells patients that they have done well in a vision test, acts as a sounding-board for their ideas or simply says 'I understand'; again, this should not be overdone or the optometrist will appear patronizing.

Counselling is therefore far from being a simple matter of telling a patient what to do: it is, rather, about helping the patient to participate actively in the consultation. Acting as an effective counsellor—putting patients at ease, drawing them out, giving information appropriately, and so on—necessitates good communication skills, which are considered in detail in the following chapter.

Stereotyping

The practitioner who accepts the need for patients to move out of the passive patient role must acknowledge that they are all different, and need treating as individuals. However, we all have a tendency to perceive others not as individuals, but on the basis of stereotyped ideas. An insight into this tendency is relevant not only to how the optometrist perceives patients, but to how stereotypes operating in the world at large (or at least, western culture) may influence vision care.

We all make judgements about people quite rapidly on the basis of first impressions. Even before words have been exchanged, we glean information from the so-called static non-verbal cues which they emit, such as facial appearance, hair and clothes. Simply by looking at someone we can guess fairly accurately how old they are, what their race is, whether they are male or female; we may gain some idea of their social class; we may find them attractive or otherwise; we may notice that the person is on crutches or has a guide dog. On the basis of such information, we build up certain expectations about the individual (that is, we attribute certain characteristics to them) and prepare to behave towards them in certain ways. The beliefs we have about people based on the categories into which we place them (such as 'elderly', 'blind', 'female') may not be unique to ourselves, but quite commonly held in society. In other words, stereotypes exist.

People are even willing to make judgements about others purely on the basis of facial appearance. Summarizing research in this area, Bruce (1988) notes that we seem to have a set of stereotyped ideas about what teachers, builders and criminals look like, and are willing to rate unknown people along such dimensions as honesty and intelligence, although such stereotypical attributions may be entirely unreliable. There is plenty of evidence, therefore, that faces invoke attributional processes which go far beyond the information given, and it has been suggested that this process may be perpetuated by stereotyped role portrayals in television and films (television advertisements often rely on stereotypes in order to get their messages across in the brief time-slot available).

Since stereotyping may lead us to make erroneous assumptions about individuals it seems worth asking why this phenomenon should exist. The underlying purpose appears to be one which runs through all aspects of perception: the need to deal economically with information by means of categorization (Aronson, 1972). If the brain were to store every instance of every item (and every person) encountered separately, it would be difficult to operate efficiently or work out general rules about how the world works (although this appears to be what Gibson's theory of direct perception, discussed in the previous chapter, implies). What seems more plausible is that when we face any new situation which cannot be dealt with at a direct perceptual level (including meeting a new person) we try to make sense of it by examining it in relation to other similar items we have met (or heard about) before, as a guide to how to react to this new stimulus. It is not being argued here that stereotyping is acceptable, but that it is a fact of life of which health practitioners should be aware and take into consideration in dealing with patients.

Treating patients as individuals is incompatible with treating them as stereotypes. Elsewhere in this book, the discussions of special patient groups provide information aimed at reducing the tendency to behave towards them in inappropriate (and perhaps offensive) ways, such as talking to the elderly as if they were children or the deaf as though they were stupid. However, this information still leaves one at the stage of considering people as members of categories, even if the perceptions are more accurate than those based on uninformed stereotypes. It is necessary to go further, and treat each patient on the basis of his or her own unique expectations and beliefs, a topic which is considered in detail in the next chapter.

While optometrists can beware the negative effects of stereotyping *vis-à-vis* their perceptions of their own patients, they cannot be responsible for the operation of stereotypes in the world outside the consulting room. There is still a need to consider them, however, in so far as they relate to vision care, and later in the chapter we will look at evidence relating to stereotyped ideas about people who wear spectacles.

The social significance of the eyes

There can be little question that the eyes have a special psychological significance for *Homo sapiens*. Human beings are largely visual creatures, as becomes all too apparent when sight is not present: the popular notion that the intact senses of the blind are more acute is a myth, and blind children seem to be at a particular developmental disadvantage because vision normally serves a co-ordinating function between the various senses (Lewis, 1987). Consideration will be given in the final chapter to psychological aspects of visual loss. However, the eyes are important not only because they subserve vision but because, as a facial feature, they play a central part in person perception: they have a role in expressing emotions, in defining who we are, and in interpersonal attraction. Optometrists must therefore give proper consideration not just to a patient's visual functioning, but to the social impact that the prescription of correctives may have.

It was noted earlier that facial appearance can evoke stereotypical responses from others, and the eyes play a part in this: for example, in one study, it was found that increasing the size of the eyes in schematic faces increased the attribution of physical weakness, submissiveness and intellectual naivety (McArthur and Apatow, 1983–84).

The eyes also serve a signalling, or communication, function, in forming a part of overall facial expression: for example, they are opened wide in surprise and fear, but narrowed in puzzlement or hostility. The 'eyebrow flash' seems to be a universal gesture of recognition and greeting (Eibl-Eibesfeldt, 1972). Eye contact is another important aspect of communication: it plays a part in communicating emotions (for example, prolonged eye contact can indicate sexual attraction or hostility, depending on other contextual cues); it also helps to control the flow of conversation (Argyle and Cook, 1976). We normally take such processes for granted, but can become aware of them when the usual systems are disrupted, as in the case of the disconcerting effect of having a conversation with someone with strabismus.

While the significance of faces has long been of interest to social psychologists it has in recent years also become a major area of interest to cognitive psychologists, who are particularly interested in the complex processes involved in recognizing faces (Bruce, 1988). After overall facial outline, the eyes are the most important feature in identifying a face (Fraser and Parker, 1986). The face is the most reliable key to individual identity, and is therefore very intricately tied up with both how others see us, and how we see ourselves—our self-image. If someone does not want to be recognized, they may use ploys such as changing hairstyle and adding spectacles, and it has been shown that such changes do indeed make someone harder to recognize (Patterson and Bradley, 1977). It is not difficult to see, therefore, how the initial prescription of spectacles could threaten self-image purely from the viewpoint of changed appearance (besides any additional meaning which may be attributed to the need for correctives, such as advancing years).

Person perception and the wearing of visual correctives

Patients may be concerned about the way they will appear to others if spectacles are worn. Is this a real issue, or are patients simply tiresomely vain? Given the foregoing evidence that the face and eyes are of special social significance, the optometrist needs to take seriously the proposition that some patients may have valid concerns relating to the social consequences of wearing spectacles. A certain amount of research has been carried out in this area, which has been labelled 'the psychology of visual correctives' or 'psycho-optometry'.

Researchers have examined the proposition that stereotypical images of spectacle wearers exist. This is important, since patients' ideas about the wearing of spectacles may be influenced by such stereotypes. Considering the much-quoted couplet penned by Dorothy Parker in the 1920s, 'Men seldom make passes/at girls who wear glasses', the influence of spectacle wearing on facial attractiveness is especially worthy of attention (Parker, 1926). This is not a trivial matter, as people really do take facial attractiveness very seriously, as witnessed by the use of cosmetics and, in some cultures, even surgery to change appearance. What is considered attractive may depend on culture (Martin, 1964), but there is a high level of agreement among western observers as to what constitutes an attractive face. A face may be judged as more attractive when the pupils are dilated (as occurs in sexual arousal), hence the use of belladonna in the past as a beauty preparation. The importance of the eyes in interpersonal attraction nowadays is indicated by a study which found that young women tend to regard their eyes as their most attractive facial feature (Terry and Brady, 1976).

It has been shown, perhaps disturbingly, that the attractiveness of one's face can affect the kind of person one is perceived to be. Attractive people are judged to have better and happier lives and to possess more socially desirable personality traits—the 'beautiful is good' phenomenon (Dion et al., 1972). This has been elegantly described by Aronson (1972):

> It turns out that our visual perception exercises a terribly conservative influence on our feelings and behaviour. We are wedded to our eyes— especially as a means of determining physical attractiveness. . .pretty people are likely to strike us as being more warm, sexy, exciting, and delightful than homely people.

Aronson went on to describe experiments in which people 'turned off their eyes', and became acquainted with one another solely through the sense of touch, and prior stereotypes were dramatically diminished.

In real life, though, we do not turn off our eyes, and the research just described indicates that patients may have good reason to be concerned about whether spectacles will influence the perceptions that others hold about the types of people they are. Is there any truth, then, in the notion that spectacles affect the way people are perceived by others? A number of studies have examined this possibility. The first studies in the area appear to be those of Thornton in the 1940s (Thornton, 1943, 1944). Using both photographs and live models, these experiments indicated that people were rated as more intelligent, dependable, honest and industrious when wearing spectacles.

Harris et al. (1982) found that fictitious people whose descriptions included the wearing of spectacles were rated as relatively intelligent, hard-working and successful, but not active, outgoing, attractive, popular and athletic; this effect occurred regardless of the sex of the described person. Other work (Edwards, 1987) has supported the notion that people who wear glasses are perceived as more intelligent and less attractive and, again, that this effect holds equally for men and women. These studies indicate, therefore, that people who wear glasses, both male and female, may be perceived differently from others in a whole range of respects as well as attractiveness.

Other studies, however, have suggested that male and female spectacle wearers are perceived differently. A recent re-analysis by Terry of an earlier study indicated that photographs of women were judged as less attractive and men as more attractive with glasses (Terry and Kroger, 1976; Terry, 1989). Terry (1989) also produced further support for the idea that male and female spectacle wearers are perceived differently, his later study improving on previous work in a number of ways. The subjects were asked to rate a stimulus person, who was supposedly being interviewed for a job, on several gender stereotypical and task-relevant traits. A woman was judged as less successful, less honest, less quick-witted and more of a follower when she wore her glasses; a man wearing glasses, on the other hand, was judged as more successful, honest and quick-witted, and more of a leader. However, the findings on attractiveness did not reach statistical significance in this study.

Experimental evidence does suggest, therefore, that how people are perceived by others is influenced by the wearing of glasses, and there is a little evidence that women may be at a particular disadvantage. In general terms, the popular notion that people with glasses are seen as more intelligent and less attractive has found some support. It is of anecdotal interest at this point that when British television cameras entered the House of Commons for the first time in November 1989, there was much discussion about the image that Members of Parliament would be projecting: it was reported that many would be attempting to read their speeches from large print, without their customary spectacles, so it appears that in British politics beauty is seen as more salient than intelligence!

A question related to the perception of spectacle wearers by others is how they perceive themselves. This question of self-image was addressed in a study which only included female subjects (Terry and Brady, 1976), the focus being on self-rating of facial attractiveness. Those who wore glasses were inclined to rate their overall attractiveness and eye attractiveness as lower than those who wore contact lenses or no correctives, and there was evidence that these women also devalued the importance of their eyes for attractiveness and emphasized other facial features. This finding fits well with the theory that people maintain high self-esteem by devaluing the importance of negative aspects of self-image (Rogers, 1951), although the finding that spectacle wearers nevertheless perceive their faces as rather less attractive suggests that the strategy is only partially successful (they may, of course, devalue the importance of overall facial attractiveness for self-image, but this was not studied).

All the above studies were carried out on young college-age people, so it is not known whether similar findings apply to other age groups. There is anecdotal evidence that the wearing of spectacles by children can cause them to be teased by peers and, if very young, pitied by adults, but there do not appear to have been any formal studies on this. It is also not known how older people respond: many people will be prescribed spectacles for the first time in middle age, and it is uncertain how this affects self-image as related to the ageing process.

Nevertheless, with regard to young adults at least, the studies mentioned have a number of implications for the optometrist. The primary one is that cosmetic considerations are likely to be high on the list of priorities for most people requiring a correction, and those faced with the prospect of their first prescription may be influenced by stereotypical images of spectacle wearers. Thus many will be concerned that their attractiveness will be reduced, although for some this may be offset by the expectation that they will appear more intelligent and successful. In deciding how best to advise a patient, the practitioner therefore needs to be skilled in ascertaining what the particular concerns of the individual are.

In view of the importance of self-image it is clearly vital for dispensing opticians to give customers the opportunity to form a clear view of how they look wearing various frames. Video and photographic techniques can avoid the situation where a myopic customer is horrified at his or her appearance once the chosen frames are glazed. The trauma this can cause should not be underestimated: one married couple quarrelled because the myopic wife (who had a distressing history of being called 'four-eyes') refused to wear her new, expensive spectacles; in the course of the argument her husband pinned her down and forced her glasses on to her face! (She was eventually successful in wearing contact lenses, persisting despite early difficulties.) Sensitivity to the importance of cosmetic factors should help to avoid cases where patients believe spectacles reduce their attractiveness and therefore do not use them when needed, or return to complain about the spectacles ostensibly on the grounds that they are ill-fitting or vision is poor with them.

The social implications of contact lenses

Although there is only slight evidence that female spectacle wearers are judged less attractive than males, according to Terry (1989) women are more likely than men to request contact lenses, and advertising often seems to be directed towards women, emphasizing both the convenience and cosmetic advantages of contact lenses (Foot, 1985–86). As already noted, glasses do tend to lower self-rated attractiveness for women (no one has yet studied this in men), so some patients for whom this is an important issue may prefer contact lenses. It is of interest, therefore to consider briefly the psychological aspects of contact lenses.

Received wisdom has it that contact lenses have a good psychological effect as wearers will be less subject to negative stereotyping associated with spectacle-wearing, and feel more attractive. There have been reports of dramatic psychological benefits (Gording and Match, 1968), but such claims have been based on anecdotal evidence or on seriously flawed experiments. One study (Terry and Brady, 1976) showed that female contact lens wearers rated their faces and eyes as more attractive than those who wore glasses, but cause and effect cannot be assumed: it could be that those who already rate themselves as facially attractive are more likely to opt for contact lenses.

Two Canadian psychologists attempted to improve on previous work, although their study was limited to a small number of young women (Hadjistavropoulos and Genest, 1988). Established measures of facial image and shyness and sociability were used, and it was ascertained that the two groups studied did not differ initially on these measures. One group changed from glasses to contact lenses, and the other was prescribed glasses for the first time. No difference on the psychological measures was found between the two groups after several weeks. The researchers said it was possible that a difference would occur in time, or would occur in the case of those who changed to contact lenses because their spectacles had particularly thick lenses. Another point of interest, not discussed at length by the researchers, is the motivation for changing to contact lenses: over half changed for cosmetic reasons, but a high proportion had other reasons, such as convenience. It is possible, therefore, that one would only expect the social advantages examined to occur in those who were dissatisfied with their spectacles cosmetically (which may or may not have been those whose spectacles had particularly thick lenses), and the lack of significant changes in the group as a whole would not be too surprising.

A final point to be noted about psychological aspects of contact lenses is the fact that many patients do not follow instructions about the use and care of their lenses. This is discussed in the following chapter, in considering the topic of patient compliance.

Conclusions

This chapter has considered a number of social psychological aspects of vision care. The patient–practitioner relationship has been discussed in the light of role theory, and it has been argued that an egalitarian relationship is appropriate within today's health care climate, with the optometrist taking on the role of counsellor. The topics of person perception and stereotyping have been considered, both from the point of view of the optometrist's perceptions of his or her patients and in relation to the images created by visual correctives. Some psychological implications of contact lenses have also been discussed.

There are other aspects of social psychology which are also of particular relevance for vision care, including communication, the beliefs about health which people hold and whether they see themselves or others as being in control of their lives and health. These and related issues are discussed at relevant points throughout the book.

References

Argyle M., Cook M. (1976). *Gaze and Mutual Gaze*. Cambridge: Cambridge University Press.

Aronson E. (1972). *The Social Animal*. San Francisco: Freeman.

Bruce V. (1988). *Recognising Faces*. Hove: Lawrence Erlbaum.

Byrne P.S., Long B. (1976). *Doctors Talking to Patients*. London: HMSO.

Canadian Association of Optometrists (1985). The role of the optometrist in health care delivery in Canada. *Can. J. Optom.*, **47**, (suppl.), 3–7.

Dickson D. (1989). Interpersonal communication in the health professions: a focus on training. *Counselling Psychol. Q.* **2**, 345–66.

Dion K., Berscheid E., Walster E. (1972). What is beautiful is good. *J. Pers. Soc. Psychol.*, **24**, 285–90.

Dodds A. (1988). *Mobility Training for Visually Handicapped People. A Person-Centred Approach*. London: Croom Helm.

Edwards K. (1987). Effects of sex and glasses on attitudes toward intelligence and attractiveness. *Psychol. Rep.*, **60**, 590.

Eibl-Eibesfeldt I. (1972). Similarities and differences between cultures in expressive movements. In *Nonverbal Communication* (Hinde R., ed.). Cambridge: Cambridge University Press.

Foot H. (1985–86). The liberated ladies? What the psychologist thought. *Optical Manage.*, Dec. 1965/Jan. 1986, 18–19.

Fraser I., Parker D. (1986). Reaction time measures of feature saliency in a perceptual integration task. In *Aspects of Face Processing* (Ellis H.D., Jeeves M.A., Newcombe F., Young A., eds). Dordrecht: Martinus Nijhoff.

Gardner A., McCormack A. (1990). The potential role of communication in developing self efficacy in the patient. Presented to 5th European Regional Conference of Rehabilitation International, Dublin, May.

Gording E.J., Match E. (1968). Personality changes of certain contact lens patients. *J. Am. Optom. Assoc.*, **9**, 266–9.

Hadjistavropoulos T., Genest M. (1988). Reconsideration of the psychological effects of contact lenses. *Am. J. Optom. Physiol. Opt.*, **65**, 814–18.

Harris M.B., Harris R.J., Bochner S. (1982). Fat, four-eyed, and female: stereotypes of obesity, glasses and gender. *J. Appl. Social Psychol.*, **12**, 503–16.

Heron J. (1986). *Six Category Intervention Analysis. Human Potential Research Project*. Guildford: University of Surrey.

Humphriss D. (1984). *Refraction Science and Psychology*. Cape Town: Juta.

Lewis V. (1987). *Development and Handicap*. Oxford: Blackwell, p. 37.

Martin J.G. (1964). Racial ethnocentrism and judgement of beauty. *J. Social Psychol.*, **63**, 59–63.

McArthur L.Z., Apatow, K. (1983–84) Impressions of baby-faced adults. *Social Cognition*, **2**, 315–42.

Miller S.C. (1989). Impact of health care trends on the practice of optometry. *Optom. Vision Sci.*, **66**, 698–704.

Parker D. (1926). *The Portable Dorothy Parker*. New York: Viking Penguin.

Patterson K., Bradley A.D. (1977). When face recognition fails. *J. Exp. Psychol: Hum. Learning Mem.*, **3**, 406–17.

Peters R.S. (1966). *Ethics and Education*. London: Routledge and Kegan Paul.

Robinson W.P. (1972). *Language and Social Behaviour*. Middlesex: Penguin.

Rogers C. (1951). *Client-Centred Therapy*. London: Constable.

Terry R.L. (1989). Eyeglasses and gender stereotypes. *Optom. Vision Sci.*, **66**, 694–7.

Terry R.L., Brady C.S. (1976). Effects of framed spectacles and contact lenses on self-ratings of facial attractiveness. *Percept. Mot. Skills*, **42**, 789–90.

Terry R.L., Kroger D.L. (1976). Effects of eye correctives on ratings of attractiveness. *Percept. Mot. Skills*, **42**, 562.

Thornton G.R. (1943). The effect upon judgements of personality traits of varying a single factor in a photograph. *J. Soc. Psychol.*, **18**, 127–48.

Thornton G.R. (1944). The effect of wearing glasses upon judgements of personality traits of persons seen briefly. *J. Appl. Psychol.*, **28**, 203–7.

Weinman J. (1987). *An Outline of Psychology as Applied to Medicine*. Bristol: Wright.

Chapter 4

Communicating with patients

Introduction

I once asked my local optometrist what the hardest part of her job was. She replied, without hesitation, 'Dealing with people'. Vision care is an essentially interpersonal process, as discussed in the previous chapter. It follows from this that communication between practitioner and patient is as vital a part of optometric practice as it is of other health-related professions.

Given that health care practitioners spend so much of their working lives communicating with patients it might be assumed that they must be good at it, but this is not necessarily the case. One review of the literature suggested that communication breakdown between doctors and patients is the rule rather than the exception (Bourhis et al., 1989), and both doctors and nurses neglect emotional issues in favour of task-oriented information (Byrne and Long, 1976). Physiotherapists and pharmacists have also been found wanting in their ability to communicate well with patients (Dickson and Maxwell, 1985; Hargie and Morrow, 1987).

Optometrists appear to have escaped the communication researchers' eagle eye so far, and many may feel quite happy that they communicate well with their patients. However, studies have also shown that health care staff may be in blissful ignorance of their shortcomings in this respect, and a high level of practitioner satisfaction with a consultation may not be matched by that of the patient. To give just one example of lack of practitioner insight, doctors may believe they spend more time listening than talking to patients, when the reverse is actually the case (Freemon et al., 1971).

The general picture given by research is that poor communication can lead to patients feeling that they receive insufficient information and that the practitioner is not really interested in them; they are also likely to show poor recall of information and advice. The practitioner, on the other hand, may fail to extract relevant information from the patient, and suffer the exasperation which results when patients fail to follow advice and prescribed treatment (this scenario is likely to be particularly familiar to optometrists with contact lens patients). In contrast with this, patients who enjoy adequate levels of communication with health practitioners are less anxious, lonely and depressed, more satisfied with treatment and more likely to adhere to therapeutic regimens (Dickson, 1989). Fostering good communication in health care therefore seems a very worthwhile exercise, and there is no reason to suppose that vision care should be any exception. Is it possible, then, to avoid the communication breakdown which seems such a common feature of health-related consultations?

Communication can be regarded as a skilful activity, and therefore as something which can be learned and improved, and evidence is accruing that communication skills training (CST) for health care workers can be successful (Dickson et al., 1989). One aspect of communicative competence is having a conceptual understanding of the processes involved, and another is being able to put techniques into practice. This account is intended to provide the conceptual background necessary for practitioners wishing to improve their consultation skills. Hopefully, it will also put the matter of patient–practitioner communication in vision care on the map and establish recognition of the need for CST to be incorporated into optometry courses.

The nature of communication

If a patient is to be viewed as more than a passive recipient of treatment, then communication must be much more than a simple process of extracting some kinds of information from the patient and pouring in other kinds. Both participants simultaneously transmit and receive messages, not all of which are overt. The nature of a communicative interaction between two people is determined by a number of factors, which have been divided into the two categories of 'situational' and 'personal' (although in reality these cannot be entirely differentiated from one another).

Situational factors include the roles demanded and the rules which pertain (such as whether the practitioner adopts an authoritarian stance or whether a patient feels it appropriate to query advice); even such physical factors as the layout of the room can be relevant for communication. Personal characteristics include the knowledge, beliefs, values, attitudes, expectations and so on of the communicators. Even the most apparently passive patients bring in certain attitudes and beliefs which will affect the outcome of the consultation. The nature of the beliefs people hold about health matters is especially relevant.

These various factors are not static: as communication proceeds, beliefs, roles and so on may be changed. Indeed, there must be changes during the course of a consultation if it is to be successful. For example, the optometrist's initial impressions of the patient may be quite wrong, and must change if the individual needs of that patient are to be addressed. Likewise, if the patient holds erroneous beliefs (for example, that wearing spectacles weakens the eyes), then the optometrist needs to know about them and try to change them.

The communicative process in health care can also be seen as purposeful and goal-directed (Dickson, 1989), and an optometrist's communicative skill can be regarded as the ability to achieve goals set during a consultation. Although the onus is on the professional to manage the interaction in as productive a way as possible, this is not to say that the optometrist must behave in a machiavellian way, angling to impose his or her wishes on the patient (although there may be occasions when strong advice is needed). It is, rather, a matter of co-ordinating the goals of the practitioner with those of the patient, modifying them if necessary in the light of information which emerges during the course of the consultation. Above all, this involves the skill of letting patients tell their stories in their own way.

Some of the optometrist's goals, such as obtaining a good history, will be fixed for all patients, while others will be specific and develop during the consultation. For example, it may be felt appropriate to initiate patching treatment for a young amblyope. However, the patient (or family) may have conflicting goals—for instance, a parent may be against the use of an eyepatch because of concern about the child's appearance. The optometrist must have the skill to uncover and deal with concerns such as this, since the patient (or parent, in this case) may not readily admit to them, but they will nevertheless have a profound effect on compliance with recommended treatment. Discovering such concerns gives the practitioner the opportunity to take them into account in giving advice and information (in the example given, the parent might be happier if the patching regimen could be limited to hours when it could take place within the home).

An important aspect of communicative skill is an awareness of the importance of covert messages: regardless of what is actually said, indicators such as tone of voice and posture carry messages about dominance and submissiveness, friendliness and hostility, interest and boredom. An ability to emit and interpret appropriately such non-verbal indicators, popularly referred to as 'body language', is therefore an important component of communicative skill (Argyle, 1988).

The nature of communication in a health care context is therefore complex. The remainder of this chapter is devoted to a more in-depth examination of a number of factors identified above as being of importance. These include health beliefs, non-verbal behaviour, history-taking, communicating information and advice, and compliance.

Health beliefs

It is all too easy to see vision care as occurring purely within the confines of the consultation, and as something which is done to the patient by the optometrist. However, as indicated by research in various medical and paramedical settings, patients are not passive entities. They bring with them certain expectations and beliefs which affect the progress of the consultation. This, in turn, can be expected to influence their future behaviour and attitudes with regard to such issues as satisfaction with the practitioner, the following of advice and future consultation patterns. Why people behave as they do with regard to their health is therefore a complex matter.

As discussed by Sanders (1989), theories about health-related behaviour have attempted to account for individual differences by drawing attention to the importance of individuals' perceptions, especially as related to health threats. The most influential model has been the health belief model (HBM; Rosenstock et al., 1959). This was proposed in the 1950s, when immunizations for poliomyelitis first became available, but everyone was clearly not rushing to have their child immunized.

Although criticisms, variations and other models have since been put forward, the HBM has been the most influential over the years, and does help to cast light on the reasons why people behave in certain ways. Why does one person make and keep regular appointments for sight testing, while another repeatedly fails to turn up? Why does one person persist in trying contact lenses despite difficulty while another quickly gives up? Why does a chemical worker risk losing his vision through not using protective eyewear? Psychological literature aimed at health professionals often approaches such individual differences in terms of personality types, but this is not particularly helpful in a practical sense. Research has suggested that the best approach is for the practitioner to determine an individual's idiosyncratic health beliefs, and good communicative techniques are necessary to do this.

The HBM has drawn attention to some important areas in which attitudes and beliefs affect people's health-related behaviour. They include triggers to action, perceived risk to health, perceived benefits of and barriers to a particular course of action and beliefs about efficacy. Below, each of these will be discussed in turn, using contact lens wear and care to exemplify them.

A trigger to action is something that cues a person to take a particular step. In the most general sense, the optometrist can act as a trigger for vision care by advertising services and sending appointment reminders to patients. There will also be triggers for more specific aspects of vision care, as when someone decides to try contact lenses because an acquaintance has passed an unfavourable comment about his or her appearance with spectacles, or when an existing contact lens patient is driven to the optometrist's after reading a 'scare' article in the media (Fontana, 1988).

Perceived risk has two components—how vulnerable a person feels to a particular condition and how severe they regard it as being. One individual may feel vulnerable to conjunctivitis resulting from contact lens wear, for example, while another does not, and one person may regard it as more trivial than does another.

A person will also be concerned with the benefits of taking a particular action. One person may regard it as a great social advantage to wear contact lenses, while another may be perfectly happy with spectacles (this may relate to stereotypical images, as discussed in the previous chapter).

There may also be barriers to taking a particular action. Contact lens use can involve some initial physical difficulty and time, effort and money must be expended on a care regimen.

Finally, there are beliefs about efficacy: whether the patient believes a treatment will work or whether he or she will be able to do what is necessary. For example, some patients may feel that they will never be able to place a contact lens in their own eye. Beliefs about efficacy are closely linked with ideas about self-efficacy, which in turn relate to where patients see control of their health as lying. Some patients believe their health is in the hands of powerful others, such as health care workers or due to chance; this is referred to as an 'external health locus of control'. Others regard their health as being under their own control, that is, they have an 'internal health locus of control' (Wallston and Wallston, 1978). It is particularly important for patients to have a sense of control and self-efficacy where self-management of a condition is concerned, and this is discussed further in the context of low vision rehabilitation in the final chapter.

All these components of health beliefs will interact to determine how a person behaves. The optometrist needs to be able to determine these various aspects of patients' beliefs with regard to their vision in order to meet their needs effectively, and also to make the patient aware of the likely benefits and barriers of different possible courses of action so that the patient can make informed decisions.

Non-verbal behaviour

In the previous chapter, it was pointed out that static non-verbal cues to person perception, based on appearance, can be misleading. So-called dynamic non-verbal cues, such as posture and voice, become an important modifying force as communication proceeds (Argyle, 1988). Such cues are particularly important in terms of the emotional content of the interaction. Non-verbal leakage may occur, whereby non-verbal behaviour, which is more difficult to control than verbal behaviour, is at variance with what is actually said; for example, a person may claim to be quite relaxed while sitting with clenched fists. A good communicator must be able to detect such covert messages.

Non-verbal cues are powerful indicators of attitudes of dominance and submission, and this is relevant to the egalitarian practitioner–patient relationship discussed in the previous chapter. There is an anecdotal example of a woman who was training as a counsellor and was amazed at how authoritarian she appeared when she saw herself on video. Non-verbal cues of dominance can destroy other efforts by the health professional to act in a counselling rather than a dictatorial role.

It certainly seems to be the case that some people are naturally good at giving out and picking up appropriate non-verbal signals, and these people are likely to be thought of as socially sensitive. Others do have more of a problem, and may unintentionally come across as withdrawn, uninterested and insensitive to others' feelings. Clearly, this is not ideal for anyone practising within the health professions.

There are a number of components of non-verbal communication. These include orientation and distance, eye contact, paralinguistic cues and body movements. The following account is intended to give a flavour only of what is a complex subject, and there is some degree of cultural variation.

The orientation of interactants to one another and their distance apart reflects the intimacy of the situation. A practitioner who sits at a great distance from patients, or behind a desk, will not be sending out signals conducive to a friendly atmosphere which encourages patient participation. Seating the patient straight in the examination chair may fuel anxiety, and another chair should be available for history-taking. Thought should be given, therefore, to the layout of furniture in the consulting room. Sitting side by side is undoubtedly friendly, but can make eye contact and the detection of other non-verbal cues difficult. Sitting opposite, or at a slight angle to, the patient, is therefore preferable.

Posture can also give clues to how willing the person is to be involved in communication: leaning slightly forward indicates a positive attitude (although leaning very far forward can indicate aggression). A patient who leans away with arms and legs crossed may be tense and unwilling to talk, and assumption of this posture may indicate that a difficult topic has been touched upon. This is, of course, a two-way business: the patient will be monitoring the optometrist as well, who will appear uninterested in the patient if such a posture is adopted.

Eye contact is another important component of non-verbal communication. It helps to regulate turn-taking: the speaker makes relatively little eye contact until the end of the utterance, then looks steadily at the listener to 'hand over the floor'. Prolonged eye contact indicates strong emotion, affection or hostility, depending upon the context, while aversion of gaze indicates anxiety or embarrassment.

Paralinguistic cues include features such as tone of voice and rate of speech. Again, they are important both for regulating turn-taking and for indicating emotion. Dropping the voice, for example, indicates a readiness to hand over the floor, while a lack of readiness is indicated by raising the voice if interrupted. On the part of the listener, the emission of so-called grunts (such as 'uhuh') encourages the speaker to continue. Mood and emotion are also indicated by paralinguistic cues; an anxious person may speak quickly, with hesitations and errors, for example.

Body movements include both facial expression and more general body movements. It has been suggested that facial expression indicates the kind of mood, such as happiness, worry or depression, while other body movements reflect intensity: at the extreme, someone may leap up and down with strong emotion, but the facial expression may indicate joy or anger. The importance of the eyes in expressing emotion was considered in the previous chapter. Hand gestures are used as an accompaniment to speech, reflecting what is said and emphasizing important points. Self-manipulative movements, such as fiddling with clothing, increase during anxiety.

It is possible for a good use and appreciation of non-verbal communicative signals to be developed. Playing back videotapes of one's own interactions is particularly useful for providing information about one's own typical non-verbal style, as in the example mentioned earlier, and the reader is advised to take advantage of any opportunity to do this. However, as pointed out by Weinmann (1987), simply becoming aware of the nature and importance of non-verbal signalling may be sufficient to help a practitioner to become more adept at detecting some of the more important covert messages which patients give.

There is perhaps one note of caution that should be given: Burnard (1989) has warned against placing too much reliance on being able to read a patient's non-verbal behaviour. There are individual and cultural differences, and body language cannot be read in a foolproof way as if one were reading a book. It is, rather, a useful guide to how a person may be feeling when considered in the total context, and when used in conjunction with other communicative techniques, such as clarification and confrontation, which are discussed later.

Taking the patient's history

Taking patients' histories is a vital aspect of health care consultations yet, as with communication skills in general, learning how to do it effectively is left very much to chance (Dickson, 1989). Simply exposing students to patients or having them attached to experienced practitioners is a largely ineffective way of training them in skilled history-taking. This is not surprising given the lack of skill detected even in experienced practitioners (Maguire, 1984). Studies of doctors, senior medical students and nurses have shown that they often neglect important areas when interviewing, or collect data in ways likely to be inaccurate and incomplete. Poor use of skills in questioning patients has been found, together with failure to exercise appropriate control over the interview and failure to check whether interpretation of what the patient says is accurate. The importance of this lack of skill is indicated by the finding that two different interviewers can extract quite different information from the same patient and end up with quite different interpretations of what the patient's problem is!

It is vital to establish a good rapport with the patient from the outset. This is helped by looking at the patient and knowing and using his or her name. Trite as it may sound, exchanging a few neutral pleasantries, about the weather or whatever, is useful for establishing rapport; it has also been shown that patients are more likely to follow a doctor's instructions if the doctor is friendly and engages in some informal discussion. This should not be overdone, however, so as not to waste the time of practitioner or patient, and so as not to give the impression of not taking the main business (the patient's vision) seriously.

Although a pro forma for recording history is a useful guide in ensuring that all necessary areas are covered, and for recording information, it should not be followed slavishly from A to Z. Initial routine questions, like name and address, can be useful for easing into the interview and continuing the process of establishing rapport. These questions, and others, such as 'When did you last have a sight test?', have fixed answers, and are known as closed questions. The dangers of asking a whole list of such questions are, firstly, that the interview may be steered down a particular alley, thus closing off other avenues for exploration and, secondly, that patients may drop into a mode of responding by only answering questions rather than being forthcoming about their own viewpoint.

The aim should be to achieve a two-way flow of communication. It has been shown with medical interviews that this is best achieved by starting off not with closed questions, but with open-ended questions, of the type, 'What did you want to see me about?'. This particular question does not seem of real value in the case of an optometric consultation, as it seems to invite the answer, 'I want to have my eyes tested'. Obviously, the difference is that a doctor needs to start by getting into the right general area, whereas the parameters of the vision test are more narrowly defined. However, there may be other, similar questions which would be useful, such as, 'Did you have a particular reason for coming to see me just now?' This gives patients the opportunity for putting across their problems as they see them.

It is advisable, however, not to put this question right at the start of the interview, but to allow rapport to build up through general conversation and during a few closed questions. This is because a patient who has a particular worry may not be willing to open up at an early stage (see Chapter 5 for a further discussion about patient anxiety). Such opening up may occur quite late, in fact, as in the situation familiar to doctors when a patient who is about to leave says, 'By the way, while I'm here. . .'. So, even if a patient claims to have simply come for a routine check-up, the practitioner should bear in mind the possibility that there may be other problems still to be ascertained. This can be approached again later in the interview, following some further routine closed questions (such as 'Is there any family history of glaucoma?'), by putting more open-ended questions, such as 'Is there anything else you'd like to discuss?' or 'Have you any queries we haven't covered yet?' A good two-way flow of communication is facilitated by the development of an awareness of the difference between closed and open questions and the achievement of a good balance between them.

If a patient becomes silent or seems to be having difficulty discussing a particular topic, the temptation is to avoid the silence and butt in with more closed questions. Paradoxically, however, in this situation, silence by the practitioner can encourage communication. It must, however, be an attentive silence, accompanied by non-verbal signals which indicate a willingness to listen to what the patient has to say. These include looking at the patient, readiness to make eye contact, looking interested and giving little nods and grunts when the patient does begin to respond.

If this strategy fails, and the patient seems uncomfortable with the silence, there are two alternatives. One is to go back to some direct questioning. The other, which can be used if there is a suspicion of an emotional response which the patient is not expressing, is to use confrontation. Despite its name, this should be in no way aggressive; it consists of the practitioner suggesting his or her perception of the patient's feelings, saying, for example, 'You seem upset', or 'You seem to be having difficulty telling me about this'. This is often enough to get the patient to say what the problem is. If not, the patient's decision not to open up should be respected and the interview should move on.

Clarification is a useful technique for ensuring understanding of the patient's viewpoint. It consists of the practitioner offering a summary of what he or she understands the patient's view to be, and offering the opportunity to correct it. This should not be overused, however, as it can give a mechanical feel to the interview, or even suggest that the patient should not add anything further (Burnard, 1989).

These techniques can be used not just to ascertain worries which the patient may have, but to determine what the patient's expectations are, such as what he or she expects to gain from the consultation, or to happen in the future.

Giving information and advice

At various points in the consultation, but particularly at the end, following the examination, the optometrist will have information to convey to the patient about his or her vision or perhaps general health; it will be necessary to try to account for any reported symptoms, and there may be certain instructions to follow: when to wear glasses, how to look after contact lenses, how to use a low vision aid, how best to present educational materials to a visually handicapped child, that referral to a general practitioner or ophthalmologist is needed, and so on.

There are a number of factors to be taken into account here. Will the patient understand what is being said? If so, will it be remembered? Will remembered instructions be followed? Finally, all these points tie up with the general level of patient satisfaction (Ley, 1988).

Firstly, then, there is the question of understanding. There is a great deal of evidence that patients frequently fail to understand medical information, for two main reasons. The first is that clinicians often present information in too difficult a form. The second is that patients bring in their own beliefs, and interpret what the practitioner says in the light of their own existing framework of understanding. Ambiguity can be a problem in this respect, and a (possibly apocryphal) story about this has been told by Pickwell (1987). The optometrist, with Maddox groove in place, says, 'Can you see the red line running up and down?' and the patient replies, 'No, It's not running up and down. It is quite still'. It has been pointed out that even simple, everyday words can be ambiguous in a medical context—consider, for example the contrasting meanings of 'tablets taken for sleeping' and 'tablets taken for pain' (Ley, 1988). The practitioner needs to look out for such ambiguities, although in practice they are likely to be difficult to spot.

Other problems can arise when the practitioner uses technical terms. In a study of general practice patients and polytechnic students, over half did not understand the term 'dilated' (Cole, 1979), which any vision care professional might use without a second thought. Humphriss (1984) suggests avoiding the word 'fixate' in giving instructions to patients, as few know what is meant. Other terms which I have seen drawing blank looks from patients include 'meridian' and 'periphery'.

Experience in Cardiff Visual Assessment Unit also indicates that very few parents know the meaning of the word 'astigmatism', and some confuse it with 'squint'. Suppose the optometrist told such parents that their baby had some astigmatism, which would be corrected at a later date if necessary. The parents might go away worrying, quite unnecessarily, about the prospect of their child needing surgery. On the other hand, being totally unable to see any sign of a squint themselves, they might go away thinking that the optometrist is totally incompetent, and would probably go else-where next time and advise their friends to do the same.

Another example from my own experience came about when I was trying to explain to a woman who had had a stroke that it was causing her problems with visual attention. She thought I meant that she was using her visual difficulties to draw attention to herself. I then realized that I had used the word 'attention' in a technical sense that would not have been familiar to her. I was horrified at the interpretation she had made, but very relieved that she had queried it.

Many misunderstandings could be cleared up if patients asked questions, as that woman did, but there is plenty of evidence that they do not often do so. Something in the region of a half of medical patients do not ask for information they want (Klein, 1979). It has been suggested that one reason is that patients often have a deferential attitude to doctors, and therefore feel inhibited. Whether they have a similar attitude to optometrists is open to question, but it is likely that some do, particularly if optometrists encourage authoritarian relationships with patients. Irrespective of this, many patients are probably simply afraid of looking foolish in displaying their ignorance. There are several consequences of this lack of question-asking: patients are less informed than they would like to be; practitioners think patients want less information than they actually do, and practitioners may overestimate their own communicative competence as patients seem satisfied (Ley, 1988). It should always be borne in mind, then, that patients may well not have understood an explanation, and plenty of opportunity should be given in a supportive way for them to ask, so that they don't feel foolish. It is useful to have some simple explanations of various points ready, such as describing the astigmatic eye as being shaped more like a rugby ball or American football than a soccer ball.

Just as there is evidence that patients often fail to understand what they have been told, so there is evidence that they often forget (although, contrary to what might be expected, there is only a slight indication of reduced recall in the over-65s). Forgetting was demonstrated in a study of 100 patients who had undergone surgery for detached retina, who recalled only about 57% of what they had been told (Priluck et al., 1979). Patients tend to remember a smaller percentage of the information the more information they are given. However, what patients do recall soon after the consultation they are likely to retain, and they are most likely to remember what they see as the most important points. It is necessary, then, to ensure that it is conveyed to patients which are the most important points. Patients also tend to remember best what they are told first, and repetition aids recall. Remembering is enhanced if the information is given using simple words and short sentences.

A technique which can help recall is categorization of the information. The practitioner might say, for example,

> Now I am going to tell you:
>   what the problem with your vision is;
>   what treatment I suggest;
>   what the outcome will be.

These headings are then filled in.

Finally, the use of written back-up information can also help recall and, just as with oral information, short, simple sentences are remembered best. Clompus (1984) is a strong advocate of the use of preprinted materials in optometric practice. He suggests that the practitioner should take note of which areas seem to create the most misunderstandings, and prepare information sheets on those topics. One he has found particularly useful is 'Normal Symptoms for First Time Bifocal Wearers', which lists and explains six common symptoms. He also recommends giving contact lens patients with chemical sensitivities a sheet listing solutions which are non-thimerosal–preserved or non-preserved. He has also produced sheets for low vision patients on topics such as macular degeneration, cataract and the use of low vision aids, all printed in large type.

Compliance

The problem of patients failing to comply with the advice of health care practitioners is such a major one that one journal, *Journal of Compliance in Health Care*, is entirely devoted to it. One study which demonstrated objectively lack of compliance was done on ophthalmological patients (Norell and Grantstrom, 1980). They had glaucoma, and had to use pilocarpine drops every 8h. These were supplied in a container which incorporated a device which automatically recorded the timing of the opening of the container. It was found that the mean gaps between doses were about 6h, 6h and 11h rather than regular 8-hourly intervals.

Compliance is a problem in optometry just as much as elsewhere. Patients fail to turn up for appointments, they wear their spectacles inappropriately and come back and complain, they return low vision aids unused, and there are many articles in optometry journals about the failure of patients to comply with instructions about contact lenses. One study found that out of 100 asymptomatic contact lens patients, more than half had care systems with contaminants, including bacteria, fungi, *Acanthamoeba* and endotoxins (Weissman, quoted in Fontana, 1988). Similarly, Collins and Carney (1986) found that only a quarter of contact lens patients were fully compliant.

Such lack of compliance, as well as creating health risks, causes bad relations between patient and practitioner, and poor satisfaction all round. It is easy, in such situations, for each party to blame the other (Heszen-Klemens, 1987). Attribution theory is relevant here: this has been developed to examine beliefs about the causation of events, and a common attribution error is to attribute negative behaviour in others to their personality, but in oneself to external influences. For example, *you* fell over because you are clumsy, while *I* fell over because the ground was slippery (Jones and Nisbett, 1972).

Applying this to the present context, Clompus's (1984) comment is relevant: 'Whether the patient is struggling with his first pair of bifocals or develops a red eye from improper contact lens care, he'll hold you responsible for his problems'. From the practitioner's point of view, blaming the patient is particularly easy, as the very term 'compliance' implies that the patient ought to do as instructed. Some workers now question the use of the word, saying it smacks of an old-fashioned authoritarian attitude by health care workers, and fails to take account of the fact that the patient also has a viewpoint to bring to the situation. The term 'adherence' is sometimes used as an alternative.

A more productive approach than blaming the patient is to analyse the situation and see where things have gone wrong and how they might be improved. The guidelines to good communication given above will indicate the possible ways in which communication breakdown may have occurred: not behaving in a friendly manner, failing to ascertain the patient's viewpoint, using technical terms without explanation, failure to categorize information and so on. This is all of especial importance if the patient has to follow complicated instructions, as is the case with contact lens use and care, since that is when compliance is lowest. It can also be helpful to look at the situation in terms of the HBM, whereby the patient's appreciation of risks and benefits, and perception of barriers to compliance help to account for whether compliance will occur. There is some specific evidence that practitioner knowledge about the HBM can improve patient compliance (Inui et al., 1976).

Another finding is that long waiting-times are associated with non-compliance, therefore an efficiently run practice is important. A related aspect here is the failure of patients to keep appointments. This has been studied for hospital, general practice and dental care, and in the region of a half of appointments are broken. The figures improve by about 20% if a postal or telephone reminder system is used. Reminders are particularly useful if the original appointment was made some time ahead. It may be partly a question of overcoming forgetting, and partly a matter of conveying that the practice is caring and efficient. Clompus's (1984) reminder cards list the date of the last visit and the purpose of the recall (routine examination, contact lens visit, etc.); in some cases a phone call is used as a final reminder. However, there must be a limit to what the practice can tolerate, and he allows patients two 'no-shows', and double-books the third appointment so that the practice does not suffer (a final resort is giving the patient a list of other optometrists in the area).

There are two interesting side-issues with regard to compliance which warrant consideration before leaving this topic. The first arises from the study of compliance in glaucoma patients described earlier. One woman was called in for interview because she was unique in taking her drops at precise 8-h intervals. It turned out that she had been carefully following her doctor's instruction that she must take the tablets exactly as directed or she would go blind. She had taken this so literally that she was terrified that she would go blind if she missed a single dose, and this had gone on for 4 years. This was described in the *Lancet* as 'malignant compliance' (Norell, 1982), so the poor patient is as damned for following instructions as for not doing so! The lesson to be learned from this is that patients need to be realistically informed about the risks and benefits of different courses of action so that they can make their own decisions.

An example from experience in Cardiff's Visual Assessment Unit is of a woman who came for a second opinion regarding patching her 2-year-old strabismic daughter. She'd been told by an orthoptist that she must patch her for a certain length of time daily or the little girl would lose the sight of the eye. As so often happens, her daughter objected so violently that the mother found patching impossible without actually pinning the girl down, and she wanted to know how important it really was. What she needed was information about the costs and benefits of patching and advice on possible ways of getting her daughter to accept the patch, so that she could then make an informed decision on the basis of her own priorities (methods recommended to encourage acceptance would be based on behavioural principles, utilizing reward and gradually approximating to the desired behaviour, as discussed in the next chapter).

The final point to make about compliance is that it is not just patients who do not comply (Ley, 1988): there is evidence that health care professionals also fail to follow proper procedures. Pharmacists omit warnings about medicines they dispense; nurses ignore hospital rules about giving medication; dentists do not give irradiation protection for their patients' testes and ovaries, and psychologists fail to follow the rules in psychological assessments. I leave it to the reader to provide examples of non-compliance by vision care professionals.

Conclusions

This chapter has pointed out the central importance of good communication skills in health care practitioners—skills which are often lacking, but can be developed. The importance of ascertaining the patient's viewpoint has been discussed, in the light of the HBM. Communication skills examined included the appropriate use of non-verbal behaviour, the use of open and closed questions, and giving information and advice in ways that patients are most likely to understand and remember. Finally, ways of encouraging compliance with—or adherence to—information and advice are outlined.

References

Argyle M. (1988). *Bodily Communication*. London: Methuen.
Bourhis R., Roth S., MacQueen G. (1989). Communication in the hospital setting: a survey of medical and everyday language amongst patients, nurses and doctors. *Soc. Sci. Med.*, **28**, 339–46.
Burnard P. (1989). *Counselling Skills for Health Professionals*. London: Chapman and Hall.
Byrne P., Long B. (1976). *Doctors Talking to Patients*. London: HMSO.

Clompus R. (1984). How I head off those poor compliers. *Rev Optom.*, February, 23–4.

Cole R. (1979). The understanding of medical terminology used in printed health education materials. *Health Ed. J.*, **38**, 111–21.

Collins M.J., Carney L.G. (1986). Patient compliance and its influence on contact lens wearing problems. *Am. J. Optom. Physiol. Opt.*, **63**, 952–6.

Dickson D.A. (1989). Interpersonal communication in the health professions: a focus on training. *Counselling Psychol. Q.*, **2**, 345–66.

Dickson D., Maxwell M. (1985). The interpersonal dimension of physiotherapy: implications for training. *Physiotherapy*, **71**, 306–10.

Dickson D., Hargie O., Morrow N. (1989). *Communication Skills Training for Health Professionals. An Instructor's Handbook*. London: Chapman and Hall.

Fontana F. (1988). Can we improve contact lens compliance? *Rev. Optom.*, February, 91–100.

Freemon B., Negrete V., Davis M., Korsch B. (1971). Gaps in doctor–patient communication: doctor–patient interaction analysis. *Paediatr. Res.*, **5**, 298–311.

Hargie O., Morrow N. (1987). Introducing interpersonal skills training into the pharmaceutical curriculum. *Int. Pharm. J.*, **1**, 175–8.

Heszen-Klemens I. (1987). Patient compliance and how doctors manage it. *Soc. Sci. Med.*, **24**, 409–16.

Humphriss D. (1984). *Refraction Science and Psychology*. Cape Town: Juta.

Inui T.S., Yourtee E.L., Williamson J.W. (1976). Improved outcomes in hypertension after physician tutorials. A controlled trial. *Ann. Intern. Med.*, **84**, 646–51.

Jones E.E., Nisbett R.E. (1972). The actor and the observer: divergent perceptions of the causes of behaviour. In *Attribution: Perceiving the Causes of Behaviour* (Jones E.E. et al, eds). Morristown, NJ: General Learning Press.

Klein R. (1979). Public opinion and the National Health Service. *Br. Med. J.*, **1**, 1296–7.

Ley P. (1988). *Communicating with Patients*. London: Croom Helm.

Maguire P. (1984). Communication skills and patient care. In *Health Care and Human Behaviour* (Steptoe A., Mathews A., eds). London: Academic Press.

Norell S.E. (1982). Malignant compliance. *Lancet*, **i**, 50.

Norell S.E., Grantstrom P. (1980). Self-medication with pilocarpine among outpatients in a glaucoma clinic. *Br. J. Ophthalmol.*, **64**, 137–41.

Pickwell D. (1987). Communication with children. *Optom. Today*, May 9, 322–3.

Priluck I.A., Robertson D.M., Buettner H. (1979). What patients recall of the preoperative discussion after retinal detachment surgery. *Am. J. Ophthalmol.*, **87**, 620–3.

Rosenstock I., Derryberry M., Carriger B.K. (1959). Why people fail to seek poliomyelitis vaccination. *Public Health Rep.*, **74**, 98–103.

Sanders L. (1989). Psychological correlates of negative self-assessed health. *Counselling Psychol. Q.*, **2**, 249–59.

Wallston B.S., Wallston K.A. (1978). Locus of control and health: a review of the literature. *Health Ed. Monogr.*, **6**, 107–17.

Weinmann J. (1987). *An Outline of Psychology as Applied to Medicine*. Bristol: Wright.

Chapter 5
Vision care through the lifespan

Introduction

Although the principle of treating patients as individuals is paramount, age can act as a rough guide to the kinds of considerations likely to be relevant for vision care. At one time, psychologists spoke of development as if childhood were the only time when important changes occur, but now broader views have come to the fore (Baltes et al., 1980). It is certainly true that particularly dramatic and rapid changes take place during infancy and childhood, and the greater part of this chapter is devoted to these early years. However, the term 'lifespan development' has now been introduced into psychology, acknowledging that people do not become set in concrete at the end of adolescence: they continue to change, physically, cognitively and in terms of their major preoccupations, problems and interests.

These changes will be under the combined influence of both the environment and biology, but the relative weight of each will depend on the circumstances; for example, while age of school entry is determined mainly by the social environment, the timing of puberty is largely under biological influence. Some changes happen to almost everyone within a society, that is, they are normative changes—starting school and reaching puberty are two examples. Other events are non-normative, such as being born with defective vision or sustaining a head injury.

Lifespan developmental psychology has brought with it a new understanding of the importance of the environment in development, both within the family and the wider social context, and the role of the family in health care is discussed at the end of this chapter. However, the individual is not being passively acted upon by outside forces, but is interacting with the environment and helping to produce his or her own development; for example, the infant actively explores and makes sense of the environment (a process that will be more difficult for the child with physical or intellectual impairments).

This chapter examines some of the changes which typically occur through the lifespan and their relevance for vision care. A useful framework for looking at lifespan changes is in terms of developmental tasks (Havighurst, 1972). These are tasks which typically arise at certain periods of life and which, if successfully completed, lead to happiness and to success with later tasks; lack of success leads to unhappiness and social disapproval and lays the foundation for further failure.

Infants

Vision and Early Development

In Havighurst's terms, the tasks of infancy include learning to walk and talk and to develop concepts and learn language to describe social and physical reality. Vision normally plays a central part in such processes.

It is not just the case, though, that infants must 'see to learn': in some respects they must 'learn to see' also. The recent explosion of interest in measuring babies' vision has resulted in part from an increased appreciation of the need to detect and remediate visual problems as soon as possible: for example, the plasticity of the human binocular system declines quite rapidly from about 2 years of age, so that late treatment of binocular problems will have limited success (Banks et al., 1975).

In addition, new methods have been developed which make the testing of such young patients possible. The most influential technique has been that of preferential looking, devised in the 1960s by Fantz and colleagues to investigate the perceptual preferences of infants (Fantz, 1961). Fantz showed that infants will spend longer looking at some patterns than others; for example, they prefer a schematic face to a face with scrambled features or no features. Infants will look at a pattern in preference to a blank alternative of equal luminance, and the acuity card technique has been developed utilizing this principle (Teller, 1979). The infant is shown gratings of increasing spatial frequency and eye movement observations are used to assess preference; acuity is defined as the highest frequency which is preferred to the grey alternative on 75% of presentations (see Lewis and Maurer, 1986, for a comparison of different psychophysical methods).

The preferential looking technique is applicable to other visual functions, such as stereopsis and contrast sensitivity. The usefulness of this is as yet confined mainly to research, although there is work in progress aimed at developing clinical tests of contrast sensitivity suitable for infants (Woodhouse. personal communication).

Assessing vision and treating problems early is important not only to prevent permanent visual impairments, such as amblyopia, but to give the child with visual difficulties the best possible chance of utilizing vision effectively in development or, if vision is so impaired that this is not possible, to enable special services for the blind to be brought into play as soon as possible so that alternative, non-visual routes to development can be fostered.

Understanding of normative life events can be enhanced by considering non-normative situations, and the importance of vision in general development has been demonstrated by studying children with severe visual impairments (Fraiberg, 1977; Lewis, 1987). They reach for objects later than other babies, may not crawl at all and tend to walk later, as there is no visual incentive to motivate such activities. Both the lack of visual incentives to action and, perhaps, a tendency of carers to do things for the child, may lead to underused hands, which Jan et al. (1977) called the 'floppy hands of the blind'. Their understanding of the world lags behind as vision normally helps to integrate information from the other senses, such as touch and hearing. They may also have language and other social difficulties; for example, they cannot observe facial expressions, and often lack expressiveness themselves. Infants with severe visual impairment will have difficulty learning by observation—in learning to feed themselves, for example, or to maintain good posture and gait.

Studies of sighted babies have also shown the importance of vision in learning about the environment from others. By the end of the first year, babies can co-ordinate their direction of gaze with that of other people, which means that attention of infant and adult is directed at the same object, which the adult will point towards, name, discuss and otherwise bring into the interaction (Collis and Shaffer, 1975).

Vision therefore normally plays a central role in early development, and the child with severely impaired vision will face special difficulties. Even relatively mild visual defects will put a child at some disadvantage. For example, an uncorrected myopic child may not realize that stars exist, or that trees have separate leaves; the hyperopic child without spectacles may seem unable to concentrate on close activities; a colour-defective child will not understand criticisms of his strangely painted pictures, while children with unclear vision may miss out socially by not quite grasping what is going on (Chapman and Stone, 1988).

The early detection of problems is therefore vital for a child's total development, even before formal education begins. Remediation may involve the provision of refractive corrections, the supply of low vision aids, referral for possible surgery or orthoptic treatment and giving relevant information to parents and others working with the child. This is especially important if the child has additional disabilities (see Chapter 7).

Infants' ability to co-operate with vision testing

Testing very young infants can prove difficult for the simple reason that they must be caught while awake and happy! The average newborn sleeps 18–20 h a day, but gradually spends more time in a state of alert inactivity, which is when a good response to testing of any kind is likely (Helms and Turner, 1981). By a month of age, the baby will be spending about 20 hours a week alert but inactive. Infants have individual patterns of wakefulness and sleep (such as being awake most of the morning but sleeping in the early afternoon). They also differ in personality right from birth, some being more fussy (and therefore harder to examine) than others (Bell, 1968), and most babies will not be particularly happy when a feed is due. Appointment times are therefore best scheduled in consultation with parents, who will know when the baby is likely to be at his or her best.

Obviously, an infant's understanding of vision testing will be severely limited, and testing depends in the main on observing responses which occur automatically to certain visual stimuli, as discussed in Chapter 2. However, many older infants (12 months or even less) can understand a simple request to find a visual stimulus (for example, in the Frisby stereopsis test, 'Where's the ball?'), and respond by looking at the target or touching it [according to Schaffer (1989), actual communicative pointing does not occur until the second year, but some infants below a year old will point at stereo targets on request: Shute et al. (1990)].

Reinforcement, or reward, can also be used to increase the frequency of a desired response. Stephens and Banks (1988) found that presenting noisy toys when a correct preferential looking response was made did not increase responding in 5–7-month-old infants, but this could have been because they were already performing optimally (attentive, easier-to-test infants were selected for the study). Reinforcement is generally effective with older infants, who are more easily distracted by their surroundings, and operant preferential looking, a technique specifically based on reward, has been developed. An example of research using this method was a study by Birch and Hale (1988) of binocular and monocular acuities; they gave toddlers a piece of cereal following each correct preferential looking response.

Infants' fears during testing

The social development of the infant is important because it affects the way in which the optometrist can relate to the baby. Babies recognize their own parents from a young age; for example, the mother's voice is discriminated from that of a stranger within only 12 h of birth (DeCaspar and Fifer, 1980). However, young babies are not usually upset by the presence of strangers. Later, however, at around 7–9 months, they become wary of strangers—a natural protective response at an age when babies are becoming mobile. It used to be referred to as a fear of strangers (Bowlby, 1969), but it is now recognized that this term is too strong: although wary of strangers, most babies will respond to them if someone to whom they are attached, such as a parent, is present (Sroufe and Waters, 1977). Vision testing of infants can take place with the child on a parent's lap, and most babies accept this quite well. It may be best for preferential looking tests to be carried out with an assistant holding the infant if possible, as parents sometimes have a tendency to turn the child towards the target, but this is unlikely to be possible with many babies who have become wary of strangers.

Sudden, unexpected happenings are fear-provoking for babies, so it is advisable to move smoothly with infants (dropping something loudly on the floor during testing can be disastrous, as I know from personal experience!). It is useful to have a dimmer switch in the testing room, so that if the lights need to be turned off the baby isn't suddenly plunged into darkness. This is also helpful with older infants, who are increasingly likely to be afraid of the dark. They also come to fear new experiences, and this includes things like patching for monocular testing and wearing red–green goggles for stereo testing (as with the TNO test). With some children, particularly between 1 and 2 years of age, patching will prove impossible, and so monocular acuity testing will not be possible. However, this is not too disastrous if a positive stereo result can be obtained (using a test such as the Lang or the Frisby, which does not require special glasses) as the presence of stereo indicates that there is no gross ocular anomaly (Shute et al., 1990).

It is also likely to be very difficult to persuade infants to wear an uncomfortable trial frame. This does not usually matter, as retinoscopy can take place quite satisfactorily with hand-held lenses (Rosner, 1982). There may be occasions, however, when a very precise retinoscopy is needed and the use of a trial frame would be desirable. The following case study from Cardiff Visual Assessment Unit demonstrates that it may sometimes be possible to persuade a young child to accept a trial frame by the application of simple behavioural techniques. The patient was a 14-month old girl who had been born prematurely, and was therefore at greater risk of visual problems, and preferential looking indicated that her acuity was below normal. A high degree of astigmatism was suspected, and the optometrist wanted to utilize a trial frame to determine the degree and angle accurately. This proved possible by shaping her behaviour (gradually approximating to the desired result), and reinforcing correct behaviour (accepting the trial frames). This was done by my holding the trial frame in front of my own eyes (earpieces towards the child) and playing peek-a-boo with her. She smiled and laughed, and I gradually came closer and closer until the frames touched her face; I then put the frames on her for a second, continuing to say 'boo', and gradually increased the length of time they were on her, saying what a clever girl she was. She accepted the frames and a precise retinoscopy was possible.

The use of cycloplegia for retinoscopy, while largely overcoming accommodation, has a number of drawbacks, including the slight but important risk of toxic or allergic reaction, the possibility of upsetting the child (which, as discussed below, has implications for later vision testing) and the subsequent impossibility of carrying out near vision tests, including using acuity cards and stereopsis tests. This latter drawback is not inconsiderable given that with infants and toddlers the testing routine needs to be flexible as the mood of the child changes. The Mohindra dark-focus technique is therefore preferable in the majority of cases (Mohindra et al., 1978).

Measuring infants' visual fields

Measuring the visual fields of infants is not done on a routine basis, but it may occasionally be thought desirable, particularly if the child has visual or other developmental problems. It is difficult to measure babies' fields using sophisticated equipment such as a bowl perimeter, as the tester is out of the baby's sight and the baby often beomes upset and shows wandering attention. Babies have difficulty in realizing what has become of hidden objects (including, presumably, people), especially if they shift from place to place (Harris, 1989), and it is in any case probably disconcerting for them to be spoken to by a dismembered voice when face-to-face contact is normally an integral part of their social interactions. Confrontation testing or a simple black arc perimeter used in conjunction with the white balls from the Stycar equipment can be successful for field testing infants under 1, as it is then possible to maintain social contact with the baby during testing (Dodd and Leat, 1990).

Children and adolescents

Developmental tasks

In terms of Havighurst's theory, children's major developmental tasks include learning to read, write and calculate, developing concepts necessary for everyday living, forming peer relationships and developing attitudes towards social groups and institutions. The educational (and later, career) implications of vision are therefore particularly important at this stage. This is also a time when the foundations of attitudes towards health care are being laid and, it is argued here, the optometrist has a part to play in developing an understanding of, and a positive attitude towards, vision care.

Most school-age children can cope with the usual adult vision testing procedures. When seeing older children, it is important to consider the relationship of their vision to school activities, including close work and sport. Some school-aged children will be brought to the optometrist because of problems at school, particularly with reading, in case they can be explained by a visual deficit; this is considered in detail in the following chapter.

Children's understanding of health and their bodies

As they grow older, children are better able to co-operate actively with testing procedures, provided a child-friendly atmosphere is established and explanations are given in a way the child can understand. It can be difficult to decide what level of explanation to offer to a child, but it is helpful to have a general idea of the way in which children's ideas about health and their bodies develop as they grow older. Just as it is now recognized that adults hold beliefs about health, illness and their bodies which can affect the progress and outcome of consultations, so it is now accepted that children have viewpoints which need to be considered.

This is quite a new area of psychological research. Many studies so far have been at a descriptive level rather than making use of statistical analyses, and the designs of some studies have not always been the best. Nevertheless, there seems to be a degree of consensus about the way in which children's understanding of health matters develops. Burbach and Peterson (1986) reviewed the literature and outlined a number of general changes which take place as children mature. Age is at best only a rough guide to what to expect, as there is wide individual variation, and the practitioner needs to talk to the child to try and gauge the level of explanation with which the child can cope.

Children who are brought for sight testing may have very little idea what it is all about. Even adults can have very vague ideas about how their bodies work, and the majority are unlikely to understand much about vision (see Chapter 8 with reference to lack of knowledge in cataract patients). The same applies even more to children, who may be completely bewildered by vision testing and its purpose. Young children's ideas about health matters often turn out to be surprisingly vague or mistaken from the adult and professional point of view. They often use external cues as to their state of health, so that 4-year-olds may know they are ill because they have been kept home from school or nursery, while 8-year-olds are more likely to describe illness in terms of how they feel. An optometrist's youngest patients are therefore likely to have great difficulty in explaining or appreciating any visual problems they have; they will probably accept them as normal, only realizing they are not if adults observe and label unusual behaviour on their part (for example, 'Emma can't see very well—she's always bumping into things').

Young children tend to overuse the idea of contagion, believing that all ills arise from contact with their surroundings or other people; a 3-year-old may say she caught a cold from the sun, for example. A young child with visual problems will have very little notion of why this should be so, and will probably not be able to understand detailed explanations. One or two studies suggest that body image can be distorted by specific illness experience, such as in the case of some children with diabetes who think they have no pancreas, or that their stomach is enormous because they must eat so much food. Some children with visual impairments or other disabilities may therefore have quite strange ideas about their own bodies.

By about 6 years old children think of their bodies in functional terms, for example, muscles help the leg to move, so explanations about their eyes helping them to see and glasses helping them to see better will be understood. There seems little harm in saying this to younger children also, but they are less likely to understand and, as will be discussed shortly, interaction with younger children should be mainly aimed at reducing anxiety. It is only towards the teenage years that most children can appreciate abstract ideas about how their bodies work, and explanations about long and short sight and so on are appropriate then. Below this age, more concrete explanations are needed, and carefully chosen metaphors may be useful at all ages (as in the example given in the previous chapter where the astigmatic eye was described as being shaped like a rugby ball).

Young children do not see their health as being in their own control, while as they grow older they increasingly do so; older children are therefore capable of, and may want a say, in what is going on. However, it is reassuring for even the youngest children to retain a degree of control over a situation. So, for example, rather than telling a 3-year-old 'Now I'm going to put a patch over your eye' it is often better to offer two patches (perhaps with different designs on them) and ask which they would prefer.

As children grow older, creating good relationships with peers of both the same and the opposite sex becomes an increasingly important developmental task. Self-image and acceptance by peers are important issues for young people, and not to be dismissed lightly. Older children and teenagers are often more concerned with the social aspects of health issues than anything else, so they may refuse to wear spectacles in case they are teased, regardless of the resultant problems in seeing. Unwillingness to wear spectacles should be less of a problem than it once was, with fashionable frames available; in fact, some children with perfect vision want spectacles. However, contact lenses may be a useful option in some cases.

Alleviating anxiety during testing

Some children are anxious about sight testing because they have had unpleasant medical experiences in the past; young children are particularly likely to overgeneralize from one situation to others (Steward and Steward, 1981). Young children and older anxious children often believe that illness is their own fault, and such ideas have probably been being reinforced by parents, who often say 'I told you so' when a child catches a cold after disobeying an order to wear a hat, or falls and cuts a knee while running, having been told to walk carefully. Some young children may therefore think any visual problems have been brought on by themselves (suppose, for example, they have a parent who keeps telling them not to sit too close to the television because it will ruin their eyes). This can lead young children not to report or to deny physical problems in case they are told off. It may also be connected with the finding that many young children believe that painful or unpleasant medical procedures are a punishment for being naughty.

Suitable, simple explanations and a child-friendly atmosphere are needed. Wilkinson (1988) has proposed that any medical consultation involving a child should have what he calls a 'moral order' similar to a play situation. In other words, there should be no sense of blame, or judging, or having to get things right, so that anxiety is alleviated and communication facilitated.

It is important to create an atmosphere which is welcoming for the child, with no white coat, and with toys and a child-sized chair or two available. As with any patient, rapport must be established, and this means including both child and parent. Health professionals often forget this, and talk to the parent only, then wonder why the child seems afraid when the examination is suddenly thrust upon him or her. Children can always be included in history-taking, even if they can do no more than give their names. With experience, it becomes possible to judge with a fair degree of accuracy from talking to the children how they are likely to respond to vision testing—when they are settled enough to begin testing, for example, and whether acuity cards, a letter-matching test or a

Snellen chart is most appropriate. Testing can be eased into from a relaxed history-taking during which the child plays with the toys, and stereopsis tests are very useful for this: it is a very small step from looking at a picture book to looking for the Lang pictures, for example.

Preschoolers respond best to medical examinations when the practitioner displays warmth—being physically close to the child, giving verbal expressions of empathy (indicating understanding of the child's feelings) and giving hugs or gifts at the end of the consultation (Hyson et al., 1982). Youngsters visiting Cardiff's Visual Assessment Unit are offered an instant photograph of themselves to take home, another is put up on a notice-board in the clinic and this is often eagerly sought out on subsequent visits. Little sticky badges for the child to wear, as often given by dentists, are another possibility.

It is very easy for health professionals to take their job so much for granted that they forget that it may be new and anxiety-provoking for some patients, particularly children. At some hospital eye departments, for example, cycloplegia is administered routinely to the children in the waiting room one after the other, and their protests are ignored, presumably on the grounds that it has to be done and so firmness is needed. In the short term, this is effective in that it relaxes accommodation. However, optometrists and orthoptists often see children who are terrified of later visits for vision care because they are afraid of drops. When a child can be assured that these will not be necessary (because of the use of the Mohindra technique) they almost always relax and become co-operative.

Research has indicated that young children are often afraid of aspects of medical procedures which seem trivial to adults, and so everything should be explained to the child (briefly and simply) as the examination progresses. Some children become very worried that trial frames are actually horrendous-looking spectacles that they are to be prescribed, so it should always be explained that they are not proper glasses, but just there to help the optometrist to check their eyes. Children (and adults) respond with less anxiety when they have been told what to expect; before ophthalmoscopy, for example, if the child is old enough to understand, it should be explained that the light will be bright, and may make their eyes water.

Similarly, if drops do have to be used, the child should not be told that it will not hurt, as this destroys trust between the optometrist and the child (Pickwell, 1987). However, words should be carefully chosen, as people tend to experience what they expect; they should not be told 'this will sting', but something like, 'this may feel a bit funny for a minute, but it will soon feel better'. (I have chosen not to suggest Pickwell's phrase that it feels a bit like getting soap in the eyes, having experienced the sheer hysteria that a bit of shampoo can cause in small children!) The child should be given a reason for the use of drops; that they help you to see into their eye is probably a close enough explanation for little ones, but older children can be given more detail, such as saying that it will relax little muscles inside the eye. Children who have been cyclopleged should also be told that things will look blurry for a while, even after they've gone home—imagine being told the optometrist is someone who will help you to see better, and yet you come out seeing decidedly worse!

A final cautionary note is that young children may not understand jokes, and take what is said quite literally, especially in a strange situation such as vision testing when they do not know what to expect. One optometrist joked to a 5-year-old, when the trial frames kept slipping, that they would have to be nailed on, which resulted in a screaming child clinging to her mother, and an equally distressed optometrist.

Health education and the optometrist

It seems reasonable to suppose that children learn about health matters through a combination of their own experience and the social meanings put on those experiences by others. This might occur informally, such as at home, in formal lessons at school or as a result of health care experiences.

We have already seen how children's earliest health-related behaviours are labelled and explained by adults, but children's attitudes towards health care soon appear to diverge from those of their families. For example, children's attitudes to dental care are at first similar to those of their mothers, but differ from them by 9 years of age; presumably other influences, such as the child's own dental experience, have become more salient by then (Humphris, 1990).

Relatively little health education takes place at primary school level, with the exception of dental care. Later, more health education is given, but it is often a thing apart from real-life experiences. For example, girls receiving rubella immunizations in their early teens are not generally given much information about it (Wilkinson, 1988), and Eiser et al. (1983) found that although most children they interviewed would have had preventive injections, they knew very little about them, half of 9-year-olds not realizing there was a kind of medicine in the needle. This state of affairs is hardly surprising when many health professionals talk *about* the child and his or her condition to parents rather than explaining anything to the child. Wilkinson has suggested that health education would be more effective if tied in with real-life health-related experiences.

The optometrist, as a primary health care provider, is in an ideal position to use vision care as a health education opportunity. Those involved in routine screening in schools could consider offering to liaise with schools on these occasions, perhaps giving little talks about vision or having a question and answer session with the children. Some optometrists may find these suggestions revolutionary, but health care in general is moving increasingly in the direction of health education and promotion, and it is interesting to note that the Canadian Association of Optometrists already lists these as components of the role of optometrist. Just two of the tasks they list are: 'to act as a community resource for vision and health care information and as a repository for literature to this end' and 'to act as a resource and to participate in the encouragement of children, young persons . . . to practise preventive, protective aspects of health care and visual processes' (Canadian Association of Optometrists, 1985).

In the light of the earlier discussion about children's health beliefs, it is clear that any health education by the optometrist, whether simply in the form of offering explanations to children during routine testing, or in the the more organized contexts just suggested, must take account of the developmental level of the children. For example, a young amblyope is unlikely to be persuaded that patching the good eye will be worth it for the sake of future vision, so persuasion has to involve behavioural techniques, such as rewards.

Testing children's colour vision

Although testing children's colour vision is not normally done on a routine basis, it is considered here because a fair amount of research has been carried out on the developmental implications of colour deficiency, and because recent work has made colour vision testing in young children more feasible.

The usual reason for testing colour vision in adolescents, using tests such as the Ishihara and D15, is for careers guidance: a colour defect may debar a person from entering or create difficulty with certain occupations such as electronics, vocational driving, graphic design and interior decorating.

In the case of younger children, one question to be considered is whether a colour defect does, in fact, affect their general development or education. There are a number of studies which do suggest an association between colour vision and education. Espinda (1971) found that colour defective children tended to have a lower school grade–point average than those with normal colour vision. In another study, Espinda (1973) found that more than the expected number of children with colour defects were referred to special programmes for the learning disabled. Grosvenor (1977) reported poorer primary school reading performance, while Dannemaier (1972) found that secondary school children with defective colour vision had more difficulty with the biology course and were poorer achievers in the subject.

Others however, have reported no asssociation between colour deficiency and school achievement. Differences in findings may be partly due to different methods used for assessing colour vision, some of which are not appropriate for children at certain ages (Hill, 1984). It cannot be affirmed with any certainty, then, that poor colour vision is associated with poor academic achievement, but there are a number of findings which are suggestive that it may be. It does seem reasonable to suppose that young children with colour defects might meet educational problems when materials are colour-coded, for example, in reading material or mathematics, when different colours of letters or blocks are sometimes used to help explain certain concepts (Waddington, 1965). Similarly, library book categories or worksheets might be colour-coded; one can imagine a colour-defective child getting into difficulties. Older children have themselves reported particular problems with maps, with coloured chalk on blackboards, with litmus paper and with reading teachers' marks on their books, and feel limited in their career choices (Carpenter, 1983).

There is also evidence that a colour defect can lead to practical problems in everyday life. Children have reported difficulty in seeing traffic lights and brake lights when cycling, difficulty with board games and snooker, in choosing clothes which match and in seeing colour television distinctly (Carpenter, 1983).

It may be that many children overcome their problems to a large extent, particularly in the case of mild defects, by using cues other than colour—perhaps using brightness or copying what other children do. It is generally said that there is no point in testing children's colour vision before the age of career choices, as nothing can be done about it. However, in view of evidence that teachers are generally unaware that some children in their classes have colour vision problems, it seems worthwhile testing early so that teachers can make allowances (for example, using shape-coding instead of colour-coding) and be less likely to label a child as stupid or careless. The child can also be helped to come to some kind of an understanding (most children questioned by Carpenter could not explain the cause of their colour defect); that counselling would be effective is suggested by the finding that children with older siblings or other relatives with similar problems adjust to their difficulties at an earlier age than eldest or only children [Waddington (1965)—

although there is the interesting converse case reported by Waddington of a non-colour-defective girl who gave colours the names allotted to them by her colour-defective twin brother!].

Even if it is desirable to screen children for colour vision defects, this has not been easy to do in the past, as the difficulty of the tasks involved often means that children with good colour vision will fail the test. The Ishihara test is most often used, the wavy line plates being used with the youngest children, but Hill (1984) has suggested that these plates are not, in fact, suitable for screening children under the age of 8. He suggests that the Ishihara letters and tests such as the D15 and the City require even more complex cognitive skills, including colour naming and problem solving, and are not suitable for screening below the age of 12.

A preferential looking based test has been devised by Pease and Allen (1988). It consists of four pseudo-isochromatic plates, and the patient has simply to look or point at the target. They demonstrated that with children aged 3–6, the percentage failing the test was in much closer accord with known adult levels of colour deficiency in comparison with the F-2 and AO-HRR screening plates.

In another study, their test was used with primary school children (aged 4–7) and compared with the Ishihara numbers and wavy lines and the City test (Sullivan et al., 1990). Surprisingly, even the youngest children made only a small percentage of errors on the City test, therefore it seems likely that Hill's analysis of the skills required is over-complex, and that the children simply treat it as a perceptual matching task; unfortunately, though, the City is not very sensitive (that is, colour defective children can pass it). The value of the preferential looking based test was again demonstrated, however, as the youngest children made a low percentage of errors on it in comparison with the Ishihara tests, and it was also effective at picking up children with colour vision defects (as indicated by their performance on the entire battery of tests). The preferential looking test also has the advantage over the Ishihara that it is quick, simple, and includes a plate for detecting tritan defects. When it becomes commercially available it will provide a quick and simple test for children of primary school age so that preventive educational interventions can be made for any children with colour defects.

Malingering and visual conversion reaction

Occasionally, one comes across a child who displays peculiar visual characteristics, such as amblyopia (which may vary in depth on different occasions), blindness (usually monocular) and field defects, all in the absence of any obvious organic causes. These visual anomalies are therefore regarded as being of psychological origin. The amount of space given here to discussing this phenomenon may seem out of proportion to its rate of occurrence; however, when it does arise it presents a difficult clinical situation, and the subject is in any case a fascinating one to consider from a scientific, as well as a clinical, viewpoint.

Two different circumstances giving rise to these visual anomalies are described in the literature. On the one hand, there is the child who wishes people to believe that he or she has poorer vision than is really the case, and this child is said to be malingering, that is, deliberately intending to deceive others into believing that there is a visual problem. Malingering has been described as 'the wilful, deliberate and fraudulent feigning or exaggeration of symptoms of illness or injury done for the purpose of a consciously desired end' (Kramer et al., 1979). Malingering is distinguished from visual conversion reaction (VCR), in which the child is said to have genuine visual difficulty and a real illness (Barnard, 1989). Other names for VCR include psychogenic amblyopia and hysterical blindness, although Freeman (1983) believed the term 'hysteria' should be abandoned because of confusion, particularly with malingering. Neither malingering nor VCR is diagnosed when any organic cause for the visual manifestations is present, although it is said to be possible for both malingering and VCR to occur in conjunction with an organic dysfunction, or to occur together. For example, Barnard et al. (1990) described visual findings in a 12-year old boy which they thought best explained by VCR in conjunction with simulated colour vision deficits.

Although the distinction between malingering and VCR sounds a plausible one in theory, it throws up a number of problems. Firstly, while it is said that they must be differentially diagnosed (Barnard, 1989), the tests advocated for detecting them are the same. They include improving vision with suggestion and plano lenses; demonstrating stereopsis despite significantly reduced monocular vision; the presence of constricted, tubular, spiral or other non-physiological fields; inconsistent and non-physiological responses to colour vision tests.

It follows from this, then, that malingering and VCR cannot be distinguished on the basis of optometric tests, and other criteria must therefore be used. The two distinguishing features are said to be whether there is conscious intentionality to deceive and whether the condition represents a true illness.

It is a very difficult task for the optometrist to determine whether or not a child is deliberately misleading for some kind of gain, but it may occasionally be possible to reveal deception. In one case, a little girl denied seeing any picture targets on the Cardiff acuity cards, but the optometrist observed eye movements towards them; when challenged by her mother the girl became upset and said, 'I couldn't see the house or the train or anything. . .', although she had not been told what pictures to expect (Woodhouse, personal communication). If a child does not admit to deception (inadvertently, as in this case, or otherwise) it is not possible for the eye care practitioner to differentiate between VCR and malingering on the grounds of conscious intentionality.

The other criterion for differentiating the two is that the child with VCR is 'ill'. Again, this is something that the optometrist is in no position to judge, as it would need a diagnosis by a psychiatrist that the child has a psychiatric illness.

At this point, it is necessary to stop and consider what the nature of VCR, as a symptom of psychiatric disturbance, is supposed to be. The idea of VCR as a psychiatric problem dates back to the work of Charcot, Freud and Janet during the 19th and early 20th centuries, Freud's writings, of course, being the best known (Sittinger, 1988). He described conversion reactions, or conversion hysteria, in which physical problems could sometimes be the result of internal psychological conflict, psychological energy supposedly being converted into physical symptoms. Evidence for VCR comes from case studies, many of which have been reported over the years. Various workers have reported that children with the condition have been found to have a range of adjustment problems or to have suffered an accident or trauma.

The problem is that the causal links between the psychological difficulties and the visual manifestations are retrospective and based on supposition. Some cases are, nevertheless, compelling, with symptoms difficult to account for in other ways. VCR in response to trauma is a case in point: there are tragic modern-day examples of women who have become, and remained, functionally blind after witnessing the murders of members of their families. Psychiatry in general, though, is open to the criticism that it is not objective and therefore not able to yield proper scientific evidence for its contentions in the way discussed in the opening chapter of this volume (Shapiro, 1982). Scientific studies have shown that psychiatric diagnoses are not clear-cut: psychiatrists often disagree about diagnoses, similar symptoms give rise to different diagnoses on different occasions, and psychiatrists from different cultures operate on the basis of different criteria.

Gittinger (1988) has pointed out that the diagnosis of functional illness or hysteria is often difficult, and a precise definition of hysteria has never been achieved. One characteristic of functional illness is that its manifestations change with social circumstances, including the expectations of physicians. In the 19th century the French physician Charcot used to demonstrate hysteria by bringing afflicted women before classes of medical students, but after his death the occurrence of such cases diminished (Ellenberger, 1970). A modern-day example of how cultural expectations can influence understanding of VCR is perhaps the conclusion of Mantyjarvi (1981) that her sample of 52 children with psychogenic amblyopia were suffering stress at the time of puberty and prepuberty. This seems to be based on the popular idea that adolescence is a time of special turmoil— a notion that has been disproved by scientific enquiry (Coleman and Hendry, 1990).

Labelling a child with a psychiatric diagnosis has another worrying feature: the problem is then squarely laid at the child's door, whereas the problem may result from a range of factors both at school and at home. Many psychologists who work with children recognize this and also work with families.

Another matter for concern is the motivation behind the wish to separate the 'illness' of VCR from malingering. There seems to be an underlying suggestion that the two should be treated differently, perhaps reflecting the 'mad versus bad' dichotomy encountered with respect to responsibility for criminal actions. Are we to regard the malingerer as 'bad' and to be condemned (words such as 'wilful' and 'fraudulent' suggest this) and the child with VCR as 'mad' and therefore deserving of a sympathetic hearing?

From the point of view of clinical child psychology, any child who displays problem behaviours is a child who is trying, however ineptly, to solve a problem (Herbert, 1987). A child who pretends to have visual difficulties may, for example, be trying to attribute reading problems to a visual cause rather than be seen as stupid. Such a child deserves help just as much as a child who displays similar signs and symptoms but appears unaware of his or her motivation.

Considering all these arguments, the distinction between VCR and malingering does not serve any useful purpose but is, rather, potentially damaging. I advocate abandoning both terms and replacing them with the single term 'functional visual difficulty', which seems to serve perfectly well without prejudging the causes in any way.

This still leaves the practitioner with the problem of how to deal with the situation when a child's visual signs and symptoms appear to have no organic cause and/or are physiologically impossible. The general methods of Barnard et al. (1990) of trying to deal with functional visual problems seem sound, although one or two aspects of their recommendations need modification. By talking in a non-condemning way to child and parent (separately, and then perhaps together) the optometrist may sometimes be able to glean some possible reasons behind the situation, such as problems at school. A report to the family doctor (and perhaps the school) should be made, but a psychiatric referral is inadvisable, for the reasons given earlier. A recommendation for psychological assessment, on the other hand, has a number of advantages: it is not presupposed that the child is 'ill'; the child is not labelled as 'the problem'; and the educational or clinical psychologist may instigate a range of investigations and interventions, involving both family and school. A possible disadvantage of recommending some kind of further help is that it may result in a sledge-hammer being used to crack what turns out to be a very small psychological nut; the optometrist may therefore prefer simply to send a report to the general practitioner without any recommendation, leaving it entirely to him or her (the family doctor probably has a wider view of the child's circumstances) to decide what to do next. The optometrist can, in any case, keep in touch with the situation by offering a follow-up vision test.

There seems little point in the optometrist trying to decide which symptoms are due to to VCR and which to malingering; as discussed earlier, it is very difficult to determine the degree to which the child is conscious of his or her problem-solving strategies, and this is in any case immaterial when it comes to recommending that the child (and family) be offered further help: it is for the child psychologist to make decisions about the degree of insight the child has and how to deal with this.

Barnard (1989) suggests broaching with the parents in a broad way the possibility of a psychological cause. This needs to be done with great sensitivity since, as pointed out by Roberts (1986), parents may resist a psychological interpretation of the child's problems. Roberts recommends using terms such as 'reactions to stress' rather than 'psychological problems' or 'psychosomatic condition'.

There is one final note of caution to be made. It is easy to use psychology as a ragbag for explaining things we cannot understand, and there is always the danger of attributing blame to the patient in this way rather than acknowledging a lack of understanding by ourselves or the profession—another example of the type of attribution error referred to in the previous chapter. It is interesting that Charcot's student Tourette denied the existence of functional hemianopia, with the sole exception of that associated with migraine—a condition now considered to be not psychological but organic in origin (Gittinger, 1988).

Adults

The Special Concerns of Adults

Given that adulthood is the longest period of life, it is interesting that until recently it was the least-studied psychologically. Among the developmental tasks listed by Havighurst (1972) for this period are selecting a mate, rearing children, managing a home, developing a career and accepting and adjusting to the physiological changes of middle age. With the exception of women who are having babies, most young adults have less contact with the health care services at this time than at any other time of their lives.

Many people in this age group will be very busy, managing careers, homes and families, and may have difficulty finding time for vision care. Humphriss (1984) reported that some will struggle to keep an appointment although they are ill, the result being an unsatisfactory refraction. Busy parents may have to bring small children along when attending for their own vision care, and having a practice geared up for child patients, with small chairs and toys and children's books in the waiting room, can be helpful in this respect. Busy lifestyles may also account for the counterintuitive finding that people in their 50s have more memory lapses than elderly people (Rabbitt, 1988); appointment reminders and written information to take home are therefore just as important for this age group as for the elderly.

The young to middle-aged adult might be regarded as the standard patient, around whom tests have largely been designed. It is for children, elderly people and those with disabilities that special conditions apply. This may not be simply because most patients are, in fact, young to middle-aged adults, but because optometrists are in this age group themselves, and it is easier to relate to those who are similar to onself. When the other person is different a greater effort needs to be made. However, as discussed in the previous chapter, even with the average patient, the possibility of communication breakdown needs to be considered and the ground-rules of good communication applied. In addition, the perceptual and social considerations discussed in Chapters 2 and 3 must be borne in mind.

In this age group, occupational vision will be particularly important [a useful reference is North (1991)]. Based on his clinical experience, Humphriss advised against the question 'What sort of work do you do?' as some patients may see this as an enquiry as to their salary level. He suggested that 'What is the nature of your work?' is a better question. In the case of a vague response, he suggested 'In what way do you use your eyes in your work?' Further detailed questioning may be necessary to elaborate on this and to alert the optometrist as to the particular aspects of vision likely to be important, such as near vision, distance vision, colour vision or eye protection.

One aspect of mid-life is reaching the realization that one is not immortal (Levinson et al., 1978), and the physical signs of ageing, such as the onset of presbyopia, may be one factor in this change of perspective. For the 40-year-old, then, the first pair of reading spectacles may have a significance beyond improving vision, and the optometrist must be sensitive to the possibility that the occasion may mark an important transitional stage in the patient's life.

Patient anxiety

This is perhaps an appropriate point to discuss further patient anxiety. As noted in Chapter 2, anxiety can affect a patient's response to vision testing, giving unsatisfactory results. The previous chapter outlined how effective communication between patient and practitioner is enhanced and patient satisfaction and compliance with treatment improved if a patient's particular worries can be ascertained and dealt with. Techniques such as open-ended questioning and using and interpreting body language appropriately are important for doing this.

It may surprise some optometrists that vision testing is anxiety-provoking for some patients. A survey by a contact lens manufacturer found that many people are more nervous about visiting the optometrist than the dentist (Shute, 1986). Humphriss (1984) suggested that all patients will be nervous to some degree, wishing to perform well, and he reported cases of patients who consumed alcohol before testing to calm their nerves and were then, not surprisingly, difficult to test. New patients may be nervous about what the whole thing will entail. Some may be worried about the prospect of spectacles ruining their self-image. Others may be afraid that their vision is deteriorating, that they will become blind or have to face an operation, or that some other health problem will be detected.

Sometimes the optometrist will have to convey unwelcome or unexpected information: that a patient has signs indicative of glaucoma, that their cholesterol level should be checked, that their child with severe disabilities displays no evidence of visual function.

If the patient does seem to be having a worrying time, or there is unwelcome news to convey, then the optometrist will need to draw on some aspects of the counselling role described in Chapters 3 and 4. It may be necessary to allow catharsis, the release of emotion. This often happens when patients begin to talk about problems they normally keep from family and friends, as in the case of the stroke patient who cried while describing her visual problems, saying, 'I never cry. It's nice to be able to stop pretending everything's all right'.

Supportive interventions are also needed with worried patients. Simply saying 'I understand' can help them to accept their problems and work through them themselves. However, false reassurance should not be given: if a situation is bad, pretending it is not may make the optometrist and patient feel better here and now, but it will be counterproductive in the long run when the hopeful expectations are dashed. So reassurance doesn't just mean saying, 'Don't worry, everything will be fine'. It means finding out what the patient's particular worries are, certainly reassuring them if their worries are unrealistic, and providing them with whatever information will help them to deal with genuine problems.

Malingering and visual conversion reaction

Not much will be detailed about this here in view of the full discussion given earlier in the case of children, as the issues are basically the same. A thorough eye examination must be carried out to exclude organic disease. The optometrist will be seeking to demonstrate that the patient's complaints are not physiologically credible, such as finding impossible visual fields or varying degrees of amblyopia at different testing distances. It may be more difficult to demonstrate such things in a sophisticated adult.

As with children, the distinction between malingering and VCR hinges on how conscious the individual is of the underlying motives but, again, this is not clear cut. As Milder and Rubin (1979) noted; 'all of the malingerer's motives may not be totally conscious and, conversely, not all the hysteric's entirely unconscious'. With adults, however, a possible motive for pretence that must be borne in mind is the desire to claim compensation for some incident through insurance. Possible indicators include a history of recent injury or pending litigation. Humphriss (1984) recommended referring the patient to the general practitioner in the usual way, being sure to keep a copy of the report in case of future litigation.

The elderly

In Havighurst's (1972) terms, the developmental tasks of the elderly (or, less prejudicially, people in late maturity) include adjusting to reduced physical strength, to retirement and reduced income and to widowhood. They also have to establish satisfactory physical living arrangements and adapt to new social roles.

Elderly people represent an increasing number and proportion of the population in western societies. For example, it has been estimated that by the year 2020 over 15% of people in the USA will be aged over 65 (Siegel, 1980). Women constitute over two-thirds of the elderly population, and nearly half of these are widows. Many elderly people, besides being in reduced financial circumstances, may be more socially isolated because of lack of money, transport or ill health.

These demographic changes have implications for health care in general, including vision care. Optometrists can expect the proportion of elderly patients to increase, and thus to see increasing numbers who are experiencing age-related deterioration in visual function, both as a result of normal changes in eye tissues and an increased incidence of eye pathology (Padula, 1982). Despite this, students of vision science are generally given little exposure to gerontological or epidemiological issues (Kline et al., 1982). Low vision is obviously a particular concern with patients in this age group, and loss of vision is considered in more detail in the final chapter. However, even those who are not experiencing drastic reductions in visual function may fear that this will occur: loss of vision has been rated second only to cancer as a dreaded consquence of ageing (Cogan, 1979).

The elderly are particularly likely to have multiple physical problems. In contrast with the young visually impaired, those over 65 with visual problems are twice as likely to have other physical or sensory impairments, such as hearing impairment, paralysis and speech problems (Kirschner and Peterson, 1979). The effects of strokes and hearing impairment are considered separately in Chapter 7. Health problems may prevent some patients from attending at an optometrist's practice, and there is a greater need for domiciliary visits in this age group. Contrary to popular images of the elderly, only a small minority are in residential care, the majority remaining at home. Making the most of their visual capacity can be an important factor in assisting them to remain independent.

Apart from sensory changes, there are changes in perception, and older people become slower and more cautious on perceptual judgement tasks. This may be partly due to cognitive slowing-down and partly due to increased caution (wishing to take time and get the answer right). This has obvious implications for vision testing, in that the elderly may be slower in responding when asked to make perceptual judgements. The optometrist needs to be patient, therefore, especially as trying to rush things will only result in the patient becoming anxious and making more mistakes (see Chapter 2).

Memory tends to become worse as people grow older but there is very little evidence that the elderly have a worse recall of medical information. However, where hearing problems compound the difficulties of processing information (Chapter 7), it may be advisable to provide written reminder materials for the patient to take home. Any patients who are known to have a particular problem with memory could have this noted on their record cards, so that a reminder telephone call can be given prior to an appointment.

Just as a child's age can only be taken as a rough guide to level of functioning, so is the same true of adults. While age is statistically associated with increasing mortality and morbidity, age in itself is a poor predictor of how any particular individual is functioning, and variability between individuals increases with age. On a non-verbal intelligence test, for example, two-thirds perform as well as younger people, with a third performing at a low level and pulling down the overall performance of the age group (Heron and Chown, 1967). As with all other groups considered in this book, then, elderly people should be treated first and foremost as individuals, with the optometrist treating the possible problems of ageing as a background of information which may or may not need to be drawn on with a particular patient.

This means the avoidance of treating elderly people in a stereotypical way. They can suffer from this in the same way as people with disabilities, and this is reflected in the way people talk to them; typically, younger people talk down to the elderly (Ryan et al., 1986). They are also likely to attribute behaviour to different causes in the young and the elderly (for example, a young person involved in a car accident may be assumed to have been speeding or drinking alcohol, while an elderly person might be seen as incapable of driving safely because of being 'past it'). It is important for health care workers to be aware of these social attitudes, since being treated as old can actually make people behave 'old', becoming literally more hunched and helpless than they need be. Lack of social and intellectual stimulation can also result in a deterioration of functioning. It is a sad fact that the health care of the elderly is often seen as a low priority, and forcing them to become old before their time may result in a downwardly spiralling quality of life.

This chapter began with a lifespan perspective. Coleman (1982) has pointed out how important this view is as far as the elderly are concerned, although it is a view which has not generally been taken in research. He has argued that we can only understand the lives, needs and wishes of elderly people by appreciating their life history—something which we can only do by taking the trouble to talk to them. The rules of good communication apply in equal force whatever the age of the patient.

The family

Just as the individual's life can be described as a series of stages, there is a typical series of events in the evolution (and eventual dissolution) of the family. Typically, the family is formed following marriage and the birth of the first child; the family extends as further children are born, then contracts as they begin leaving home. Dissolution occurs with the death of one spouse (World

Health Organization, 1976). Of course, this is an over-simplification: many couples have children without marrying, there are increasing numbers of one-parent families and of divorces and second marriages, resulting in step-families. Neither does a family really end when an elderly spouse dies: adult children will still interact with the remaining parent in most cases, although this can be difficult with increased mobility in employment, resulting in the moving away of adult children from their home town. Frequently there will be a role-reversal later in life, with children taking care of parents' needs rather than vice versa.

The family can be seen as a background against which the individual operates. In reality, the health care professional rarely works with isolated individuals. Parents bring children for vision testing, adult children accompany elderly parents and even the adult who comes alone will be bringing in beliefs influenced by the family and will probably go back and discuss with them what has transpired. Some patients may even attend for vision care simply because they have been forced into it by the family (Shindell, 1988).

Numerous studies have indicated the influence of the family on health beliefs and health behaviour. We saw earlier how very young children's health beliefs are influenced by the labels adults give to their behaviour, and how dental attitudes in the under-9s are related to those of parents. Haynes et al. (1979) looked at a large number of factors, over a range of studies, to see how they related to compliance. Health beliefs were important, and so was the influence of friends and family. Health beliefs themselves are influenced by friends and family, and Tuckett et al. (1985) have noted that this influence, the 'lay referral system', can over-ride that of medical opinion.

The importance of family influence on health care has also been shown by studies on children with diabetes whose condition has to be managed at home by the family. Marteau et al. (1987a) showed that the adequacy of metabolic control was related to family psychological functioning, parents' marital relationship and family composition. Marteau et al. (1987b) also showed that the treatment goals of doctors and parents often differ, resulting in conflict over management of the child's condition. They recommended that treatment goals should be made explicit so that any differences in opinion can be aired. This underlines the importance of good communication skills in finding out the point of view of patients and their families and of giving advice in a way which which is understood and remembered.

The practitioner–parent relationship can be particularly prob-lematical when the child has disabilities and often becomes adversarial in nature. Seligman and Seligman (1980) have identified five negative attitudes which the professional may assume and which can lead to a scenario of conflict. These are feeling pity, fear or hostility towards child or parents; feeling hostile or hopeless about the situation; reinforcing the family's denial of the problem; viewing patient or parent observations as untrustworthy or meaningless; viewing patient or parents as emotionally disturbed.

Other chapters in this book indicate ways of avoiding or overcoming such difficulties. The guidelines on good communication will help the optometrist to find out about and deal with the particular concerns of the family. A background understanding of various disabilities and a knowledge about suitable vision testing techniques will dispel feelings of fear or hopelessness.

The problem of dismissing parents' observations about their child is a very real one. An example from Cardiff's Visual Assessment Unit makes the point well. A 13-year-old girl was brought for visual assessment by her parents. She had been blinded in an accident at the age of 5, attended a school for the blind and read by means of braille. Her parents and teachers had become increasingly convinced that her vision was returning in one eye, but this possibility had been repeatedly dismissed by ophthalmologists on the grounds that it was not possible in view of the medical condition, and the parents reported feeling labelled as fussy and overhopeful. However, her functional vision had never been assessed. Using both acuity cards and the Cambridge letters (which only involve matching, not naming, letters) we found a corrected acuity of 6/45, albeit with very restricted visual fields. Her teacher had enquired whether any sighted reading work was a possibility, so we sent her the results of the assessment, together with an indication of the print size she would be able to see.

At the other end of the age-scale, Milder and Rubin (1979) have emphasized the role of the family in assisting patients in adjusting to aphakia. They point out that the frightened candidate for surgery may not register the information given, so the family can be recruited and given information in advance to assist in postoperative orientation.

Families, then, are an inevitable influence on patients. However, as the examples given above suggest, the practitioner need not see them merely as a necessary evil, arguing with professional opinion and placing obstacles in the way of compliance, but as potential partners in aiding patients to carry through vision care programmes at home.

Conclusions

This chapter has outlined the changes that typically occur through the lifespan in terms of developmental tasks, from infancy to old age. The role of vision at different stages in life was outlined, and special considerations likely to be of relevance for the vision care of patients at various life stages discussed. Topics covered included the development of children's health beliefs, assessing colour vision in young children, alleviating anxiety and dealing with functional visual difficulty. Finally, the role of patients' families in vision care was considered.

References

Baltes P.B., Reese H.W., Lipsitt L.P. (1980). Life-span developmental psychology. *Ann. Rev. Psychol.*, **31**, 65–110.

Banks M.S., Aslin R.N., Letson R.D. (1975). Sensitive period for the development of human binocular vision. *Science*, **190**, 675–77.

Barnard N.A.S. (1989). Visual conversion reaction in children. *Ophthalmic Physiol. Opt.*, **9**, 371–8.

Barnard N.A.S., Birch J., Wildey H. (1990). Concurrent visual conversion reaction and simulated colour vision defects in a 12-year-old child. *Ophthalmic Physiol. Opt.*, **10**, 391–3.

Bell R.Q. (1968). A reinterpretaion of the direction of effects in studies of socialization. *Psychol. Rev.*, **75**, 81–95.

Birch E.E., Hale L.A. (1988). Criteria for monocular acuity deficit in infancy and early childhood. *Invest. Ophthalmol. Visual Sci.*, **29**, 636–43.

Bowlby J. (1969). *Attachment and Loss* vol. 1. *Attachment*. London: Hogarth Press.

Burbach D.J., Peterson L. (1986). Children's concepts of physical illness: a review and critique of the cognitive developmental literature. *Health Psychol.*, **5**, 307–25.

Canadian Association of Optometrists (1985). The role of the optometrist in health care delivery in Canada. *Can. J. Optom.*, **47** (suppl.), 3–7.

Carpenter D.V. (1983). An examination of the difficulties encountered by colour defective children in a Wiltshire school. MEd thesis, University of Bristol.

Chapman E.K., Stone, J.M. (1988). *The Visually Handicapped Child in Your Classroom*. London: Cassell.

Cogan D.G. (1979). Summary and conclusions. In *Special Senses in Aging* (Han S.S., Coon D.H., eds). Ann Arbor: University of Michigan Press.

Coleman J.C., Hendry L. (1990). *The Nature of Adolescence*. London: Routledge.

Coleman P.G. (1982). Ageing and social factors. In *Psychology for Physiotherapists* (Dunkin E., ed.). London: Macmillan/British Psychological Society.

Collis G.M., Shaffer H.R. (1975). Synchronization of visual attention in mother-infant pairs. *J. Child Psychol. Psychiatry*, **16**, 315–20.

Dannemaier W. (1972). The effects of color perception on success in high school biology. *J. Exp. Ed.*, **41**, 15–17.

DeCaspar A.J., Fifer W.P. (1980). Of human bonding: newborns prefer their mothers' voices. *Science*, **208**, 1174–6.

Dodd C.G., Leat S.J. (1990). The assessment of visual fields in infants. *Ophthalmic Physiol. Opt.*, **10**, 411.

Eiser C., Patterson D., Eiser J.R. (1983). Children's knowledge of health and illness: implications for health education. *Child: Care, Health Dev.*, **9**, 285–92.

Ellenberger M.F. (1970). The Discovery of the Unconcious: the History and Evolution of Dynamic Psychiatry. New York: Basic Books.

Espinda S.D. (1971). Color vision deficiency in third and sixth grade boys in association to academic achievement and descriptive behavioral patterns. *Dissert. Abstr. Int.*, **32**, 786.

Espinda S.D. (1973). Color vision deficiency: a learning disability? *J. Learning Disabilities*, **6**, 163–6.

Fantz R.L. (1961). Visual preference and experience in early infancy: a look at the hidden side of behavior development. In *Early Behavior* (Stevenson H.E., Hess E.H., Rheingold H.L., eds). New York: Wiley.

Fraiberg S. (1977). *Insights from the Blind*. London: Souvenir Press.

Freeman R.D. (1983). Emotional components in paediatric ophthalmology. In *Paediatric Ophthalmology* vol.II (Harley R.D., ed.). Philadelphia: W.B. Saunders.

Gittinger J.W. (1988). Functional hemianopsia: a historical perspective. *Surv. Ophthalmol.*, **32**, 427–52.

Grosvenor T. (1977). Are visual anomalies related to reading ability? *J. Am. Optom. Assoc.*, **48**, 510–17.

Harris P. (1989). Object permanence in infancy. In *Infant Development* (Slater A., Bremner G., eds). Hove: Lawrence Erlbaum.

Havighurst R.J. (1972). *Developmental Tasks and Education* 3rd edn. New York: David McKay.

Haynes R.B., Taylor D.W., Sackett D.L. (1979). *Compliance in Health Care*. Baltimore: John Hopkins University Press.

Helms D.B., Turner J.S. (1981). *Exploring Child Behavior*. New York: Holt, Rinehart and Winston.

Herbert M. (1987). *Behavioural Treatment of Children with Problems*. London: Academic Press.

Heron A., Chown E.M. (1967). Age and Function. London: Churchill.

Hill A.R., (1984). Defective colour vision in children. In *Progress in Child Health* vol. 1. (Macfarlane A., ed.). Edinburgh: Churchill Livingstone.

Humphris G. (1990). Parental and child health beliefs, attitudes and behaviour. In *Psychology and Health Promotion* (Shute R., Penny G.N., eds). Cardiff: British Psychological Society, Welsh Branch.

Humphriss D. (1984). *Refraction Science and Psychology*. Cape Town: Juta.

Hyson M.C., Snyder S.S., Andujar E.M. (1982). Helping children cope with checkups: how good is the 'good' patient? *Child. Health Care*, **10**, 139–44.

Jan J., Freeman R., Scott E. (1977). *Visual Impairment in Children and Adolescents*. London: Grune and Stratton.

Kirschner C., Peterson R. (1979). The latest data on visual disability from NCHS. *Visual Impairment Blindness*, **73**(4), April, 151–3.

Kline D., Sekuler R., Dismukes K. (1982). Social issues, human needs, and opportunities for research on the effects of age on vision: an overview. In *Aging and Human Visual Function*. New York: Liss.

Kramer K., La Piana F., Appleton B. (1979). Ocular malingering and hysteria: diagnosis and management. *Surv. Ophthalmol.*, **24**, 89–96.

Levinson D.J., Darrow D.N., Klein E.B., Levinson M.H., McKee B. (1978). *The Seasons of a Man's Life*. New York: A.A. Knopf.

Lewis T., Maurer D. (1986). Preferential looking as a measure of visual resolution in infants and toddlers: a comparison of psychophysical methods. *Child Dev.*, **57**, 1062–75.

Lewis V. (1987). *Development and Handicap*. Oxford: Blackwell.

Mantyjarvi M.I. (1981). The amblyopic schoolgirl syndrome. *J. Paediatr. Ophthalmol. Strabismus*, **18**, 30–3.

Marteau T.M., Bloch S., Baum, J.D. (1987a). Family life and diabetic control. *J. Child Psychol. Psychiatry*, **28**, 823–33.

Marteau T.M., Johnston M., Baum J.D., Bloch S. (1987b). Goals of treatment in diabetes: a comparison of doctors and parents of children with diabetes. *J.*

Behav. Med., **10**, 33–48.

Milder B., Rubin M.L. (1979). *The Fine Art of Prescribing Glasses Without Making a Spectacle of Yourself.* Florida: Triad.

Mohindra I., Held R., Gwiazda J., Brill, J. (1978). Astigmatism in infants. *Science*, **202**, 329.

North R.V. (1991). *Work and the Eye.* Oxford: Oxford University Press.

Padula W.V. (1982). Low vision related to function and service delivery for the elderly. In *Aging and Human Visual Function* (Kline D., Sekuler R., Dismukes K., eds) New York: Liss.

Pease P.L., Allen J. (1988). A new test for screening colour vision: concurrent validity and utility. *Am. J. Ophthalmol. Physiol. Opt.*, **65**, 729–38.

Pickwell D. (1987). Communication with children. *Optom. Today*, May 322–3.

Rabbitt P. (1988). Social psychology, neurosciences and cognitive psychology need each other (and gerontology needs all three of them). *Psychologist*, **1**, 500–6.

Roberts M.C. (1986). *Pediatric Psychology.* New York: Pergamon.

Rosner J. (1982). *Pediatric Optometry.* Boston: Butterworths.

Ryan E.B., Giles H., Bartolucci G., Henwood K. (1986). Psycholinguistic and social psychological components of communication by and with older adults. *Lang. Commun.*, **6**, 1–22.

Schaffer R. (1989). Early social development. In *Infant Development* (Slater A., Bremner G., eds). Hove: Lawrence Erlbaum.

Seligman M., Seligman P.A. (1980). The professional's dilemma: learning to work with parents. *Except. Parent*, **10**, 511–13.

Shapiro D.A. (1982). Psychopathology. In *Psychology for Nurses and Health Visitors* (Hall J., ed.). London: Macmillan Press/BPS.

Shindell S. (1988). Psychological sequelae to diabetic retinopathy. *J. Am. Optom. Assoc.*, **59**, 870–4.

Shute R. (1986). 'It's worse than going to the dentist'. Identifying and dealing with anxiety in optical practice. *Optical Manage.*, 10–12.

Shute R., Candy R., Westall C., Woodhouse J.M. (1990). Success rate in testing monocular acuity and stereopsis in infants and young children. *Ophthalmic Physiol. Opt.*, **10**, 133–6.

Siegel J.S. (1980). Recent and prospective trends for the elderly population and some implications for health care. In *Second Conference on the Epidemiology of Aging* (Haynes S.G., Feinleib M., eds). NIH publication no. 80969. Washington, DC: US Dept. of Health and Human Services.

Sroufe L.A., Waters E. (1977). Attachment as an organisational construct. *Child Dev.*, **48**, 1184–9.

Stephens B.R., Banks M.S. (1988). Effect of reinforcement on infants' performance in a preferential lookng acuity task. *Am. J. Optom. Physiol. Opt.*, **65**, 637–43.

Steward M.S., Steward D.S. (1981). Children's conceptions of medical procedures. In *Children's Conceptions of Health, Illness, and Bodily Functions* (Bibace R., Walsh E.M., eds). San Francisco: Jossey-Bass.

Sullivan J., Shute R., Westall C. (1990). Colour vision testing in children. *Ophthalmic Physiol. Opt.*, **10**, 412–13.

Teller D.Y. (1979). The forced-choice preferential looking procedure: a psychophysical technique for use with human infants. *Infant Behav Dev.*, **2**, 135–53.

Tuckett D., Boulson M., Olson C. (1985). *Meetings Between Experts: An Approach to Sharing Ideas in the Consultation.* London: Tavistock.

Waddington M. (1965). Colour blindness in young children. *Ed. Res.*, **7**, 236–40.

Wilkinson S.R. (1988). *The Child's World of Illness.* Cambridge: Cambridge University Press.

World Health Organization (1976). *Statistical Indices of Family Life.* WHO Technical Report series 587. Geneva: WHO.

Chapter 6

Optometry and children's reading difficulties

Introduction

With increasing frequency, optometrists are becoming involved in the remediation of reading difficulties, particularly those of children. The level and type of involvement varies internationally. For example, in the USA perceptual training for learning problems is a well established practice, while optometric involvement in this area in the UK is more recent, and largely focuses on dyslexia, or specific reading difficulty. The various theories and forms of therapy that have been developed are frequently surrounded by storms of controversy, and it can be difficult for optometrists to know what stand to take amid the bombardment from commercial interests, media hype and scientific disagreements.

It is not an issue which any optometrist is likely to escape entirely, with hopeful parents bringing their children for sight testing and asking advice about the relationship between visual problems and difficulties at school. A little knowledge can be dangerous, and there have been unfortunate instances when parents and children have suffered great anguish as the result of well intentioned, but misinformed, advice from optometrists. Not only is it advisable, therefore, for optometrists in general to be well informed in this field, but some may consider the possibility of offering a specialized service in this area. Any practitioner contemplating this needs to be fully informed about the relevant arguments and pitfalls.

Dyslexia

Defining Dyslexia

The word dyslexia is one that is frequently used with reference to people who have severe reading difficulties. Developmental dyslexia, or difficulty in learning to read, is the focus of this chapter.

However, it should also be noted that people who have had a brain injury in later life sometimes have impaired reading ability, and this is known as acquired dyslexia or alexia. Attention has been drawn to similarities between these two situations, and evidence from both types of problems has been used in trying to develop models of how reading normally takes place.

Dyslexia is a topic that has aroused a great deal of controversy over the years. One definition is that it is 'a disorder manifested by difficulty in learning to read despite conventional instruction, adequate intelligence and sociocultural opportunity' (World Federation of Neurology, 1968). This is an exclusionary definition: the emphasis is on what it is not rather than on what it is, although there is an underlying assumption that the difficulty is caused by some kind of central nervous system problem.

Another approach is to regard dyslexia as unexpected difficulty in learning to read. This is another exclusionary definition, because if there is a possible alternative explanation for poor reading performance, such as low IQ, then the diagnosis of dyslexia is ruled out.

A rather different view—that dyslexia is a syndrome—has been developed by Miles (1987). His view is that the reading problems do not occur in isolation, but are associated with a range of other difficulties, including spatial difficulties, lateness in beginning to walk or talk, clumsiness and difficulty in rapidly processing symbolic material. His Bangor Dyslexia Test investigates a number of factors such as ability to distinguish left from right, to recite tables and to repeat digits. Taking into account age norms on the various items, the testee is diagnosed as dyslexic or not depending on the number of items on which he or she rates dyslexia-positive (it is usually he, in fact, as males with dyslexia outnumber females by about 3 or 4 to 1). At one time, Miles and his co-workers thought it was possible that children with dyslexia might have problems in processing visual material, but later rejected this idea, believing that their difficulty is associated with lexical coding processes: in other words, they have difficulty related to the *naming* of both visual and verbal information. So Miles has shifted away from an exclusionary definition towards a positive definition of dyslexia, but one which rules out visual problems as a cause.

Evidence relating to the nature of dyslexia was reviewed in 1987 by Snowling and by Vellutino. They reached similar conclusions, that the evidence suggests that dyslexia is a linguistic problem due to a deficit in phonological decoding ability. What that means, very briefly, is this: within an alphabetic writing system such as English, a child has to be able to deal with the correspondence between spoken sounds and their symbolic representation, and to be able to segment the stream of spoken sound into its components in order to develop literacy. There is, then an emphasis on phonology, or speech sounds. This view takes into account the finding that people with dyslexia are not just poor readers, but poor spellers, and spelling problems often persist even when reading difficulties have been overcome.

What is interesting about these two reviews is that they are so different in terms of the views of dyslexia which they considered. Snowling took a cognitive developmental perspective, based on the changes in children's linguistic skills as they mature, and how these interact with the demands of acquiring literacy; she barely referred to visual processing in her entire book. Vellutino, on the other hand, devoted his (shorter) review to debunking the idea that dyslexia results from some kind of visual problem.

The differing slants of these two reviews perhaps reflects a cultural difference. Snowling works in the UK, where the prevailing views are of dyslexia as a syndrome or as a cognitive linguistic problem; alternatively, one meets the view, particularly amongst educationalists, that there is no such thing as dyslexia, or at least, that labelling a child as dyslexic is unhelpful. In the USA, where Vellutino works, there is a tradition that reading difficulties often stem from visual problems, with optometrists playing a part in remediation.

In direct contrast with this analysis of transatlantic cultural differences is the view of Pollatsek in a review just a few years earlier (1983); he noted that the predominant view in the USA was of dyslexia as a linguistic problem, in contrast with the view then being promulgated in the UK by Pavlidis (1981) that oculomotor problems are a significant cause of dyslexia. This indicates the lability of the situation, as the influence of different theories waxes and wanes. The field currently seems as wide open as ever, with cognitivists and visualists still locked in mortal combat.

So, to return to the question, 'What is dyslexia?', the answer, which may seem unhelpful, is that it depends what any particular writer means by it. Those who believe it to be of cognitive linguistic origin would say that a child whose reading difficulties can be accounted for by some kind of visual problem is not dyslexic. Pollatsek concluded that the term refers to 'a fascinating unsolved problem for the researcher rather than to a disease entity which is well understood'. This may be almost as true today as it was in 1983, but it is not particularly helpful for the child with the problem, nor for the eye professional who has been approached for advice. Pollatsek did note, though, that there is a fair degree of consensus that what is under consideration here are children whose reading ability is at least 2 years behind what would be expected for their age. In this chapter, then, I shall use the word 'dyslexia' quite loosely to refer to children with this general level of reading difficulty, without presupposing the causes of the problem. Indeed, one of the major problems in trying to make any sense of the literature is that different writers use the word in different ways and their populations of dyslexics are by no means uniform nor, indeed, always fully defined.

The cognitive developmental view of dyslexia

The cognitive developmental view of dyslexia is the one which probably currently holds the greatest sway amongst psychologists, and a great deal of careful research in a number of areas lies behind this view. As mentioned earlier, people with acquired dyslexia have also been studied, and information gained from the two populations used, together with experimental studies of reading and of children's developing reading-related skills, to build models of how reading and spelling are normally achieved. Researchers whose work has contributed include the following (a sample reference is given in each case): Morton (1969); Coltheart (1980); Frith (1981); Bradley and Bryant (1983); Ellis (1983); Marshall (1984); Snowling (1987). Below is a very much simplified account of some of the basic features of the cognitive developmental view of dyslexia.

In learning to read, a person builds up an internal store of words, or lexicon, which can be drawn upon. However, this whole-word route to reading cannot be used when a new word, not yet in the lexicon, is encountered. Then, the word must be analysed into its component letters and matched with the corresponding speech sounds (phonemes), as in 'c-a-t spells cat'. This may be done quite literally, aloud, as when a child is learning to read, and also by some people who have had strokes which destroy their ability to access the whole-word lexicon. It may also happen quite automatically, something we can appreciate by reading a word we have not seen before: 'cobe'. This is a plausible non-word. You have never seen it before, but will automatically have analysed it into its components and applied the known rules of English to pronounce it to rhyme with 'robe'. Now read this non-word: 'stough'. You may have hesitated, wondering whether it should rhyme with 'bough' or 'enough'. Such words are irregular, and cannot be read by the analytical route; they must be learned and stored in the lexicon.

Normally, both the whole-word route and the analytical route are available when reading, although it is possible that individuals characteristically use one route in preference to the other. It is not clear how far children develop their own strategies and how far they are influenced by different teaching methods, some of which emphasize whole-word recognition while others take an analytical approach.

Either route to reading may become unavailable as a result of a stroke, giving rise to characteristic problems. In the example mentioned earlier, the person is forced to read letter by letter, having lost the whole-word route, but the reverse situation can occur, with the analytical route being lost, so that the person can only read known words, available in the lexicon, and cannot tackle new ones. Snowling (1987) has identified a similar problem in some children with dyslexia, indicated by their particular difficulty in reading non-words. She calls this 'phonological dyslexia', as it is related to difficulty in associating letters on the page with their corresponding speech sounds. This analysis can also account for the great spelling problems which are characteristic of dyslexia, as it is not possible to spell a word without the ability to translate speech sounds into their corresponding letter representations. Bizarre spellings are common in dyslexia, examples which have been reported including 'tatin' for 'traffic' and 'hisokder' for 'instructed' (Snowling, 1987).

Such children may have an underlying difficulty in analysing speech into its component sounds. It has been shown that the ability to segment sounds at an early age is a good predictor of later reading achievement, while children who are poor at this but who receive special help, with rhyming games and so on, avoid the later problems with reading. Although much remains to be discovered about the cognitive characteristics of individual dyslexic children, the general point which seems to emerge from studies is that dyslexic children have specific problems with verbal memory, verbal labelling and other aspects of auditory processing; they do not have the phonological skills required to learn to read at the critical time.

For the developmental cognitivists, then, the evidence points very strongly to phonological rather than visual difficulty, lying at the root of developmental dyslexia, and this theory can account for spelling as well as reading problems. So where does this leave the notion of dyslexia as a visual problem?

Is dyslexia a visual problem?

As will be discussed in detail later in the chapter, there have been many suggestions over the years that dyslexia results from visual problems of various kinds, such as oculomotor sequencing problems, vergence problems, scotopic sensitivity and perceptual problems.

Over the years, Vellutino (1987) has been one of the strongest opponents of the view that dyslexia results from visual problems. He showed experimentally that disabled readers can perceive letter and word symbols accurately, but mislabel them in oral reading because of a basic difficulty in associating symbols with their verbal counterparts, as described in the previous section. For example, reading disabled children were presented with words very briefly, and were just as able as normal readers to write them down even though they made more errors in pronouncing them. The findings suggested that a child who reads 'was' as 'saw' or 'b' as 'd' perceives the symbols perfectly well, but has difficulty in labelling them. Other studies by Vellutino and his colleagues showed that reading disabled children were able to perceive symbols as well as normal readers when the meaning was removed: the symbols used were Hebrew, with which the subjects were unfamiliar.

Vellutino has also argued on theoretical grounds that dyslexic children do not have visual perceptual problems, and these arguments will be discussed later in the chapter.

Findings such as Vellutino's suggest strongly that dyslexic readers are as visually capable as good readers. However, they often report visual difficulties when trying to read, and we will now consider at some length the evidence for and against various types of visual dyslexia that have been proposed.

Scotopic sensitivity syndrome

In 1983, in an unpublished manuscript, Irlen claimed to have identified a specific visual dysfunction as a major factor in dyslexia. It has been claimed that 60% of those with reading difficulties suffer from scotopic sensitivity syndrome (Clayton, 1987), and that symptoms can be dramatically improved by the wearing of individually prescribed tinted spectacles. Since then, the Irlen Institute has developed from its Californian origins to become an international commercial enterprise based on the assessment and remediation of the syndrome (which, for convenience, will be abbreviated to SSS in this discussion). Professional and lay persons receive training in prescreening, that is, in identifying likely sufferers for referral to the Institute for further testing and the provision of tinted lenses. There has been a great deal of criticism and confusion surrounding this therapy and the theory behind it, not least because much of the supportive literature remains unpublished and is therefore not readily available for scrutiny.

From a purely academic point of view, therefore, it is tempting to dismiss the whole thing out of hand, particularly as the published evidence is persuasive that dyslexia is unlikely to result from visual problems anyway. However, I believe the issue should be given proper consideration, partly on the grounds that there could be something in it—so-called crank remedies for various conditions do sometimes become scientifically respectable—and also because of the great clinical influence which Irlen's work has had. Many optometrists find themselves approached for advice on this matter, and therefore need to be aware of the issues involved.

What is scotopic sensitivity syndrome?

As all optometrists know, scotopic vision refers to vision at low levels of luminance, resulting from the functioning of the rods (Millodot, 1986), and scotopic sensitivity is measured in terms of threshold, the minimum intensity of light which can be detected (Brown, 1986). However, what Irlen refers to as scotopic sensitivity appears to have little to do with this, the central feature of the syndrome being that sufferers are said to respond dysfunctionally to specific wavelengths of light. Photopic sensitivity syndrome would therefore perhaps be a more appropriate name for the purported condition. Sufferers are said to report that, when they attempt to read, the letters on the page jump about, blur, spiral or disappear. Irlen has created a wide range of tints for spectacle lenses, and prescribes a specific one for each individual, which is said to produce sharper, clearer and more stable vision by eliminating those wavelengths to which the person responds dysfunctionally.

Irlen contrasts SSS with theories that dyslexia is a central nervous system phenomenon, but also differentiates it from such visual dysfunctions as refractive errors, muscle imbalance and difficulties with vergence and accommodation. Instead, she identifies it as a dysfunction which occurs once the image has been focused on the retina. Clayton, director of the Irlen Institute in London, states that 'full spectral light produces overstimulation of the retinal receptors which, in turn, can cause problems in seeing'. This begs many questions, such as 'which retinal receptors?' and 'what is meant by overstimulation?' No kind of physiological or psychophysiological evidence has been presented to back up this kind of statement. The picture has been further confused by Murphy's contention in an unpublished manuscript that SSS is, after all, a central nervous system phenomenon. However, his claims about the underlying genetic and cortical mechanisms (for example, that it is 'clearly found as a dominant gene on chromosome 15' and results from a 'lack of neural inhibition in the left-occipital region') are totally without foundation (Shute, 1991). Similarly, Clayton (1987) states that an individual is 'born with the condition, and it does not improve or deteriorate with time', although there have been no experiments on young babies nor longitudinal studies. Although there is evidence which suggests that dyslexia is hereditary, and that the brains of people with dyslexia differ from those of normal readers, it is far from conclusive, and relates to dyslexia in general, not to SSS.

Irlen and her supporters say that SSS cannot be detected in normal optometric or ophthalmological examinations. Her original paper said that the Irlen Differential Perceptual Schedule (IDPS) tests for problems in six categories—visual resolution, depth perception, sustained focus, span of focus, peripheral vision, and eye strain—but precise definitions are not given and how they are assessed is not explained. In Stanley's (unpublished) account of Irlen's work the six listed areas of difficulty no longer include peripheral vision, but an additional problem is mentioned— intolerance of bright light and glare (Irlen had mentioned this in her paper, but it did not appear to be covered by the IDPS). No evidence relating to the validity or the reliability of the IDPS has been presented, and the lack of detailed information about it means that Irlen's work cannot be replicated.

Studies on reading with coloured filters

Although the nature of SSS is not at all clear, the possibility exists that filters may, in some way, affect reading peformance in dyslexia. There are several published reviews of the the available evidence, all highly critical in tone (Rosner and Rosner, 1987; Howell and Stanley, 1988; Reeves, 1988; Shute, 1991). Some examples of the many problems identified are given below.

Firstly, the results of Irlen's original study were only given in subjective, qualitative terms, so that the validity of her conclusions cannot be checked. Also, importantly, between the two administrations of the IDPS an unspecified number of subjects received not just tinted lenses but changes in prescription for the correction of refractive errors; some who reported benefiting from the spectacles may therefore have done so as a result of this rather than from the tints.

Other papers supportive of Irlen, but mainly unpublished, are also seriously flawed in terms of experimental detail and design (Saint John, 1986; Robinson and Miles, 1987; Murphy, unpublished manuscript; Stanley, unpublished manuscript). Stanley, for example, used a very biased questionnaire to ascertain subjects' reactions to using Irlen lenses (for example, asking 'Has your reading rate *improved*? Has comprehension *improved*?'), thus biasing their answers in a positive direction, and of course, it would have been much more persuasive if she had measured reading rate and comprehension objectively. Some of the statements she makes are incomprehensible: for example she describes one symptom of SSS as 'parts of written work having different problems with shades of black to grey'.

One unpublished study (Winter, 1986) does seem to have included proper control groups, but has been criticized on the grounds that general conclusions about reading ability may not be drawn from it because a proof-reading task was used. However, this sort of task is very useful as it gives a quick measure of both reading rate and error rate; it does provide a good test of Irlen's proposition since, if Irlen lenses improve reading by producing a more clear and stable image, then this ought to work in the case of both reading and proof-reading. In fact, Winter found that children diagnosed as suffering from SSS read no better with Irlen lenses than with untinted plano lenses, grey lenses or no lenses.

Another unpublished paper (Adler and Atwood, 1987) claims to have supported the value of Irlen lenses, but the experimental subjects had additional treatments, including group counselling, which could account for the reported improvements in reading. Similarly, another report of improved reading performance in dyslexic children when using coloured overlays (Gregg, 1988) could be due to a placebo effect. The same applies to another study (Chelva et al., 1986) in which children's reading speed improved with their prescribed Irlen lenses. Placebo effects will be discussed further later in the chapter. Gregg's study also suffers from the disadvantages that the results were not analysed statistically and that the particular reading test used is printed on coloured backgrounds which would have interacted with the overlays. If steps were not taken to deal with this, and the children still read better with the filters, it would strengthen the suggestion of a placebo effect, and would certainly be evidence against the conceptualization of SSS as being due to dysfunctional responses to specific wavelengths of light.

One argument that can be made is that most studies are not a true test of the effect of coloured lenses on SSS, since the subjects were not pretested for the existence of the syndrome. This is necessarily so if Irlen's testing procedure is not made available for public scrutiny, and that is the catch–22 of research in this area.

The available studies, then, simply do not provide adequate evidence to support or to refute Irlen's views, but it is at least clear that she has made claims for which there is no evidence. Rosner and Rosner (1987) have called for her and her supporters to release information and funds to enable unbiased investigations to be carried out. Reeves (1988) suggests that we should not throw the baby out with the bathwater, that better evaluative studies are needed, and that even a placebo effect would be interesting. Howell and Stanley (1988) are also prepared to believe that the Irlen treatment might work in some way, but that there is no need to postulate a special syndrome of scotopic sensitivity. These points about other possible mechanisms are discussed further below, after considering one further study.

This was an undergraduate psychology project carried out by Richardson (1988). She found that the reading performance of dyslexic boys improved with a red overlay. This differs from other studies in finding that reading accuracy improved with the same filter throughout the sample, rather than with individually preferred filters, so a child might say he could see best through a blue filter, but still perform better with the red one: clearly, this militates against a placebo interpretation.

Richardson's study was well controlled: it dealt with order effects; there was a clear control filter; to eliminate practice effects, different reading passages of matched difficulty were used; importantly, reading performance was assessed blind—it was tape-recorded, and rated by judges naive to the purpose of the experiment. Richardson also borrowed Irlen's pre-screening test to confirm that her subjects probably suffered from SSS as defined by Irlen. It is unfortunate, therefore, that the filters, borrowed from the Institute, varied not just in wavelength but in transmittance, and the red filter transmitted the lowest percentage of light. It is a possibility, therefore, that the dyslexic boys were sensitive to glare from the page. This possibility has been pointed out by both Shute (1991) and by Wilkins (1990), although if this were so, neutral density filters should be as effective as coloured ones, and Winter's study on proof-reading found no improvement with any filters. Glare phenomena do not appear to be well understood, and it is only recently that attention has been given to developing methods for measuring disability glare (e.g. Abrahamsson and Sjostrand, 1986), so this is perhaps an area for future research.

Wilkins (1990) has reported that the majority of clients at the Irlen Institute choose reddish-brown tints, reminiscent of Richardson's finding with overlays. Wilkins has suggested that filters of this wavelength may be effective in reducing flicker from fluorescent lights, which seem to cause visual problems for some people. Another suggestion is that dyslexics are sensitive to the particular frequency of 'grating' which black print produces on a white page, and that reddish spectacles attenuate this problem.

Another aspect of vision which might be related to Irlen's claims is colour perception. It is strange that colour vision per se is not mentioned by Irlen, since individuals said to have abnormal retinal responses to specific wavelengths of light might be expected to have problems with colour perception (see Chapter 5 for a discussion of colour deficiency in education and testing for colour defects in young children).

So far, however, these suggestions are largely speculative, and the only solid evidence is that many people with reading problems claim greater comfort with tinted spectacles.

Implications for clinical practice

Reports of disturbing visual symptoms in connection with dyslexia, such as letters jumping and swirling about, are not confined to discussions about SSS, but have been mentioned in connection with work on lack of eye dominance and dyslexia, as discussed below. Howell and Stanley (1988) have discussed the possibility that certain conventional eye problems might give rise to such symptoms: blur and fatigue might result from accommodation problems, and fixation problems might cause letters to jump about. This is not to say that such problems *cause* dyslexia, though, as they may result from it. Irlen, of course, denies that the symptoms of SSS are caused by such factors, and emphasizes that the problems of SSS cannot be dealt with by routine optometric or ophthalmological procedures. However, since her evidence for this statement is non-existent, clearly the first course of action for the optometrist when seeing a dyslexic patient is a thorough conventional examination to check for such problems.

The possibility that the Irlen treatment might help on occasions through a placebo effect should not be overlooked. It is easy to dismiss such effects as not real, but they are: it just means that the treatment works through psychological rather than other channels. Academic achievement is not just a reflection of a child's cognitive abilities, but the product of a complex interaction between cognitive and social processes (Shute and Paton, 1990). There is evidence that a child's academic achievement is influenced by the attitudes of teachers and the attitude of the child towards his or her own ability. A child who experiences more difficulty than normal in learning to read, for whatever reason, is likely to be labelled as lazy or stupid, perhaps by the adults and children around, or by him- or herself, leading to a downward spiralling of motivation and achievement. It is quite possible that the prescription of special spectacles would break this spiral, by leading to changes in attribution regarding the child's poor academic performance: the child is no longer 'stupid' or 'lazy' but has a 'visual problem'. Quotations from Stanley's paper indicate the likelihood of this happening in the case of Irlen lenses: 'she has a confidence in her schoolwork now which has never been there before' . . . 'all the teachers are a lot nicer to me now and try to help me'.

Is this an argument for recommending the Irlen treatment? Is it ethical to recommend or prescribe a treatment because a patient wants it, or because it might have a placebo effect, even if the practitioner does not believe in it? Such treatments fall into the category of what Miles (1988) has called 'brussels sprout therapy', which will be discussed further at the end of the chapter. I advocate telling patients, quite frankly, that the scientific evidence for the value of tinted lenses is very thin, but that some people find them helpful, or restful for the eyes, and a coloured overlay will be just as effective and much cheaper. It is worth noting at this point the comment of the headmistress of a school for children with severe reading problems, that after a week or two children who have been prescribed tinted spectacles rarely use them. This suggests that any psychological benefits may be short-term, which is an additional argument for not encouraging people to go to the expense of SSS screening and prescription.

Eye movements and dyslexia

Some workers have suggested that oculomotor difficulties are a significant cause of dyslexia. This has been examined by studying eye movement patterns during reading. While reading a line of print, normal readers show a consistent series of rightward saccades each followed by a fixation, interspersed with an occasional and typically leftward saccade, or regression. This pattern is interrupted regularly with a large amplitude leftward saccade (return sweep) which marks the beginning of reading the next line of print. The primary researcher in this field was Pavlidis (e.g. 1981), who found that children with dyslexia show an increased tendency to make multiple and often large-amplitude regressions, exhibit greater variance in both the duration of fixations and the amplitude of saccades, and produce inaccurate return sweeps characterized by multiple saccades.

A chicken-and-egg argument arises here, however, as it could be that the reading problems cause the eye movement aberrations rather than the other way round. However, Pavlidis (1983) reported that these unusual eye movement patterns were not related to the level of difficulty of the reading material, as objectors to his theory would predict, and were not observed in slow-to-learn but non-dyslexic subjects. He contended that eye movement abnormalities play a critical role in dyslexic reading difficulties. Offering some support to this causal view were studies showing that subjects with oculomotor problems (slow saccades, oculomotor dyspraxia, saccadic oscillations and nystagmus) also have significant difficulties in reading (e.g. Hartje, 1972).

However, many of the studies on abnormal eye movements have been case studies or have used small numbers of subjects, and therefore say nothing about the general population of dyslexic people. Although some workers have reported the prevalence of abnormal eye movements in dyslexic subjects to be high, others have suggested that it is quite low. These disputes may have arisen partly because of differences in defining samples of dyslexics.

That eye movements are a causal factor in dyslexia has been disputed by Pirozzolo (1983), who argued that the problems were related to reading overly difficult material with a heavy linguistic load; the linguistic problems caused the abnormal eye movements, not the reverse. He quoted evidence from both normal subjects and patients with brain disease and brain damage which suggested that their abnormal eye movements were a function of cognitive processing. Abnormal eye movement patterns are also found in young children who are not fluent readers and in adults reading unfamiliar text, such as a foreign language. Also, unusual patterns occur occasionally in normal readers, suggesting that they play an insignificant role in the problems of the person with dyslexia.

Some studies have removed the linguistic element in an attempt to isolate the oculomotor component. Pavlidis (1981) did this by using small lights, sequentially illuminated in a horizontal row for the subject to follow; he found that those with dyslexia made many more regressive eye movements, with an overall increase in the number of saccades. He concluded that these differences were due to disability in sequential oculomotor control. However, subsequent similar research failed to confirm this, good readers and dyslexics were indistinguishable on the basis of their eye movements (Stanley et al., 1983).

In 1988 Raymond et al. carried out a study on the fixational, rather than the saccadic, component of reading eye movements. They examined fixational stability in 6 dyslexic children (of average or above average intelligence, but 2 years retarded in reading) with mild-to-moderate cerebellar dysfunction, as indicated by at least two signs such as impaired finger-to-nose co-ordination and gaze-evoked nystagmus. They compared them with 6 age-matched controls, using infrared recordings of their eye movements. They found that the children with cerebellar signs had abnormally poor fixational control. They acknowledged that this could be due to attentional lapses, but said that this was counterindicated by the finding that saccadic latencies when the targets moved were comparable in the two groups. Movement of the image more than 1° from the foveal centre or retinal image movement exceeding 2° substantially degrades visual resolution, so the fixational instability they demonstrated could impair visual processing during reading. However, they admit that the data do not demonstrate a causal connection between reading disability and oculomotor control deficits, so it cannot be concluded that some kind of optometric training is called for to improve reading. Also, they recognized, the findings may be limited to those with cerebellar dysfunction and may not occur in other children with dyslexia. A further drawback of the study is that the experimentals and controls were not sex-matched; most dyslexic children are male, as in this study, but most of their controls were female.

Just as with SSS, then, the role of eye movements in dyslexia has resulted in a great deal of dispute. A major difference, however, is that this debate has taken place through the pages of books and journals, with experimental details fully described and open for proper scientific scrutiny. It seems that some dyslexics do have problems with oculomotor control during reading, but not at a substantially higher level than in good readers. However, it cannot be concluded that where there are eye movement problems these cause the reading problem. On the contrary, there is a good deal of evidence that cognitive and linguistic factors affect eye movements rather than the reverse. There seem to be scant grounds, therefore, for offering some kind of training of reading eye movements for children with dyslexia.

In addition, in normal optometric practice, even if it were thought worthwhile to offer eye movement recordings, this would be impractical because of the time and equipment required. However, in Cardiff's well equipped Visual Assessment Unit we have occasionally measured dyslexic children's eye movements both during reading and when following non-linguistic computer-presented targets. This has been in response to specific requests from parents who were familiar with Pavlidis' work. If eye movements appeared abnormal, we informed the parents that the direction of causality was open to question, but if they were normal we were able to offer reassurance. In one case, for example, a boy's parents thought that he found it easier to move his eyes from right to left than from left to right, but we were able to show that he was equally capable of moving his eyes well in either direction. In this specific case it would have been particularly difficult to see how saccadic eye movements would be causing a problem, as the boy's difficulties were so severe that he was still struggling at the stage of trying to identify individual letters at the age of 8.

Binocular stability and dyslexia

Eye dominance and dyslexia

The debate about saccadic eye movements has in recent years given way to equally heated discussion about the role of vergence eye movements in reading, and their relationship to ocular dominance. The interest in this originated with Orton's (1937) suggestion that dyslexic difficulties may arise when different cerebral hemispheres control the preferred hand and the preferred eye (cross-laterality).

There are three common ways of defining the dominant eye (Porac and Coren, 1978): the eye used in monocular situations when there is a choice, as in looking down a telescope; the eye used to line up sight on a distant target, such as when pointing, or aiming a gun; the eye with the better visual acuity or without a squint. Studies using tests of monocular sighting dominance have produced no strong evidence that cross-laterality is more common in people with dyslexia.

Dunlop et al., (1973) felt that monocular sighting dominance was inappropriate when considering reading, in which both eyes are used to view a foveal target. They adopted Ogle's (1962) term 'reference eye', applicable in binocular situations, and developed the Dunlop test to determine which eye is used as a reference for the calculation of visual direction. In this test, two fused monocular targets are viewed through a synoptophore, and the tubes slowly diverged. One target will appear to move while the other remains static; the static target indicates which eye is being used as a reference. Using this test, Dunlop et al. reported a higher incidence of crossed control (with the reference eye on the opposite side to the preferred hand) in poor readers.

Stein's work on fine vergence control

Stein and his associates went on to claim that it was not crossed laterality which was related to children's reading difficulties, but whether a fixed reference eye had developed at all. This is logical, they stated, since the crossing of fibres from the retina at the optic chiasma ensures that information from each eye reaches both hemispheres (Riddell et al., 1987).

They reported that children with reading problems often say that their visual world becomes unstable when they try to fixate small letters: these seem to blur, swim around and jump over each other so that the child cannot determine their proper order (Stein et al., 1987). Stable visual localization requires that the retinal image of what is being foveated is accurately associated with ocular motor signals which indicate the direction in which the eyes are pointing at the time. Stein et al. (1987) suggested that the lack of a stable reference eye causes confusion about visual direction, so that the letters on the page appear to jump about.

This hypothesis was originally developed after studying over 1000 normally reading and dyslexic children using the Dunlop test. If there is inaccurate vergence control the child is unable to make reliable judgements as to which of the two monocular targets is being moved. The consistency of response is recorded over 10 trials. Around two-thirds of dyslexic children gave inconsistent responses, compared with just under a half of normal readers.

Increasing numbers of normal readers developed stable control with age, but fewer of the dyslexics did so. This leads again to the question raised by Pavlidis' work: does better eye movement control lead to better reading, or does better reading lead to better control?

Stein and Fowler (1985) went on to examine whether acquiring fine binocular control leads to easier reading. Monocular occlusion was used, with the aim of eliminating any physiological diplopia and, perhaps, improving fine vergence control. Half of their dyslexic subjects were assigned plano spectacles and half monocularly frosted spectacles for reading and close work. To eliminate a placebo effect or experimenter bias a double-blind experimental design was used: the children did not know which type of spectacles was supposed to be effective, and the experimenters carrying out the Dunlop test did not know which children had worn which spectacles.

Following 6 months of monocular occlusion, about a half who initially had unstable vergence control acquired stability, compared with about a quarter who had worn plano spectacles. Most with occlusion also improved in reading (nearly a year's gain in 6 months), while the plano wearers who had not gained control regressed (their reading age improved less than 6 months during the 6-month period). At the end of 6 months, the planos were changed to monocular occlusion for 6 months; 43% acquired good binocular control, and their reading improved by just over 12 months in the whole year. A third of the children with dyslexia already had stable vergence control; half of these received monocular occlusion, which slightly impeded their reading progress.

In all, the study was interpreted as indicating that up to about a third of dyslexic children can be helped to read by gaining good binocular control by means of monocular occlusion. The experimenters felt it was probably causal, as the reading improvements followed rather than preceded the binocular improvements.

The Dunlop test has come under criticism, however. Newman (1988) demonstrated that the proportion of good readers and spellers with unstable Dunlop responses was as high as poor readers; this suggests that the Dunlop is of no real value in investigating children with reading difficulties. Also, the Dunlop requires children to report their perceptual experiences—a difficult task, which means that there is likely to be a high error rate confusing the results.

Stein et al. (1987) conceded that the Dunlop was not ideal, but reported similar results using the more objective method of eye movement recordings. These indicated that two-thirds of dyslexic children were unable to make accurate vergence movements, making conjugate movements instead, leading to diplopia. This was not found to occur at all in younger children with the same reading age. However, a third of dyslexics had normal vergence control. These were said to make reading errors that were best explained by phonological mistakes, rather than by visually based ones.

Bishop (1987) offered a critique of Stein's work, refuting a number of predictions from his theory. Firstly, children with unstable dominance should be poor readers, according to the theory, but a review of studies suggested that performance on the Dunlop is a function of age and intelligence, with no evidence of a specific link between unstable performance and reading level when these variables were accounted for.

Secondly, there should be a greater prevalence of unstable vergence in the dyslexic population, but the published evidence is highly contradictory. There may be a real association in large populations which include those with the most severe problems, but this does not indicate causality.

Thirdly, the evidence relating stability of vergence to types of reading errors (visual or phonological) was not convincing. Rather, Stein and Fowler's (1985) data demonstrated that many dyslexic children with an unfixed reference eye have verbal difficulties that extend beyond reading, since at least half made phonological errors, and a substantial proportion had a history of early language delay.

Newman (1987) also reanalysed Stein and Fowler's (1985) data and directly compared treated and non-treated children, finding that the differences in amount of reading progress were not statistically significant. There was a significant relationship between the development of stable vergence and improvement in reading, but this was explicable in terms of initial reading ability: the children who developed stable vergence control in the first phase of the study tended to be those whose initial reading problems were less severe.

Stein (1987) in turn replied to these criticisms, referring to an earlier study by Bishop, which suggested that children with poor vergence and poor reading tended to have lower IQs. However, he claimed, the intelligence test used penalizes poor readers; poor vergence control could cause them to score badly. He also said that he never claimed that those with unstable reference will not show verbal deficits—many children will have both verbal and visual difficulties. With regard to the re-analysis, he criticized this for using a blunt scoring system which concealed real improvements in reading after monocular occlusion. Stein and Fowler (1985) were well aware of the problem that children with higher intelligence improved their vergence control, and in previous studies had used statistical techniques to control for this and demonstrate that reading improvement was independent of initial reading age and performance IQ (a non-verbal measure of intelligence which should not be affected by vergence problems).

Fowler et al. (1988) also carried out a study which demonstrated the importance of using small fusional targets (approximately 1°) in determining whether there is a stable reference eye, since larger targets did not differentiate between children with dyslexia and normal readers. They used this as an argument against those who have found no differences in visual performance between dyslexic and control children on visual tasks with no linguistic component, such as Vellutino's study using Hebrew symbols. The lack of differences may have resulted because large non-foveal stimuli were used.

It is difficult to draw firm conclusions about this work as yet. Certainly, Stein seems to have come up with good arguments against many of the criticisms that have been levelled at his work, and there is more work in progress relating unstable dominanace and types of reading errors. Some practitioners are already adopting this work as a basis for remedial work, using monocular occlusion (Masters, 1988), and some who favour the cognitive developmental view of dyslexia are prepared to believe it is possible that vergence problems play a small part in the reading difficulties of a small number of children.

It would be mistaken to place too much reliance on monocular occlusion therapy, as even Stein admits that it only helps a relatively small proportion of children with dyslexia. However, even this would be worthwhile for the children concerned. Perhaps carefully monitored occlusion therapy can do little harm, provided it is first established by objective means (eye movement recordings) that the child has not developed a stable reference eye; again, this suggests that it is not something which is likely to be undertaken routinely in optometric practice because of the equipment required. Such therapy should also be used only as part of a programme such as that described by Masters, where there is full co-operation with remedial teachers, educational psychologists and speech therapists, since the child is likely to have additional problems.

It also seems obvious that if some dyslexic children are indeed having a problem which is specific to foveal-sized targets, then they should find it easier to read with large-print materials. I am not aware that this has been examined experimentally, but it is usually the case that children are taught to read with flash cards and books with large print, in which case the problems which Stein claims to occur in some children should only become apparent when the children progress to smaller print.

Perceptual training for learning problems

Testing and remediating perceptual skills

Vision training is a well established practice, particularly in the USA. A child who is deficient in some aspect of functional vision, such as binocularity, vergence, accommodation, saccades and perception, is prescribed exercises aimed at improving the deficit. Particularly in the case of perceptual difficulties, the training is instigated not simply to improve visual functioning per se, but to improve the school performance of a child who is experiencing academic difficulties. Unfortunately, as discussed by Herrin (1985), vision training in general has flourished in the absence of proper scientific evidence that it is effective. In this section, the evidence with relation to perceptual training will be discussed.

Training children in perceptual skills, both visual and auditory, has been considered appropriate for learning disability—that is, for general academic failure rather than for dyslexia. The term 'learning disability' usually refers to children who have great difficulty in learning in the normal classroom context. They may be considered as having special needs or, to use an older term, to require remedial teaching, although they are not usually regarded as intellectually impaired (see Chapter 7).

One of the foremost names in perceptual training has been that of Frostig (1961). She devised her developmental test of visual perception (DTVP) after analysing various types of perceptual skills in which she found children with learning problems to be deficient. The five areas examined by the test are: eye–motor co-ordination; figure–ground discrimination; shape constancy; position in space, and spatial relationships. The child performs a number of paper-and-pencil tests of these skills, and is compared with age norms to find which areas are causing difficulty. Frostig devised a special training programme involving exercises to improve those skills which are poorly developed. However, Vellutino et al. (1977) argued that the subtests of the Frostig are so highly correlated with one another (e.g. Sabatino et al., 1974) that there seems to be little rationale for having remediation training aimed at each separately.

The work of Rosner (1979) has also been influential. He has developed tests of visual and of auditory analysis skills suitable for the optometrist to use. The visual analysis test (TVAS) is very similar to the spatial relationships element of the Frostig. The child is shown a matrix of dots, some of which are joined by lines to make a pattern; the child is asked to copy the design on to a similar, empty matrix. Increasingly difficult designs are used, and the child's ability to perform the task is compared with age norms. Children with reading problems characteristically perform poorly on this type of task, and remediation involves working on copying designs, either using paper and pencil or by stretching elastic bands on a peg board. The fact that Rosner's programme only concentrates on one area of skill in comparison with Frostig's five should not matter, given the evidence that they are all closely related anyway.

Rosner's test of auditory analysis skills (TAAS) looks at the child's ability to segment words into their component sounds. For example, the child is asked to say 'cowboy' and then to repeat it without the 'boy'. Again, there are age norms against which the child can be tested, and a remedial programme aimed at developing auditory analysis skills.

Criticisms of perceptual skills training

Larsen and Hammill (1975) criticized this perceptual training approach to the remediation of academic problems. They reviewed research on the relationship of various aspects of perceptual skill to primary school learning (usually standard achievement tests). The areas they examined were visual discrimination (such as figure–ground discrimination), spatial relations (such as might be tested by paper and pencil mazes), auditory-visual integration (for example, where the child must match sounds to dots and dashes) and visual memory.

They looked at 60 correlational studies. Of these, only 7 were longitudinal, following up the progress of individual children, and the results of these were contradictory. Also, only 6 attempted to control for intelligence. While the evidence suggested small but definite relationships between some of the types of skill and academic achievement, none was of a size that would enable academic performance to be predicted from visual–perceptual skills. They amalgamated the findings from studies which had used the same tests, and found that performance on the DTVP was correlated with arithmetic ability at an acceptable level; this remained true when IQ scores, available for a few studies, were allowed for, although chronological age was not taken into account. In general, though, they found little evidence that early visual perceptual skills are predictive of later academic achievement.

Another type of evidence that can be considered is whether there are differences in perceptual skills between high and low achievers. This is often reported to be so, but such studies have not allowed for IQ differences. Hammill et al. (1974) did so, and found no difference in perceptual skills between good, average and poor readers. They concluded that a large percentage of children who perform adequately on tests of visual perception experience difficulty in school learning, while a large percentage who do poorly have no learning problems. They recommended that the time and expense devoted to vision training in schools should be re-evaluated if the purpose was to improve academic achievement.

Rosner, despite having published a book on the remediation of visual and auditory analysis skills, later admitted that, although there are well established correlational relationships between perceptual skills and school achievement, the cause-and-effect link-up is less well established (Rosner and Rosner, 1986). In fact, Hamill and Larsen's analysis demonstrated that such correlations are generally small. The Rosners went on to suggest that only children who are slightly behind at school are likely to benefit from perceptual training alone, and older children will also need remedial help because of missing out educationally for longer.

Elsewhere in this chapter it has been noted that Vellutino was critical of vision-based approaches to learning problems, on the basis of experimental findings. He has also criticized perceptual skills training on theoretical grounds (Vellutino et al., 1977). Such training operates on the premise that perceptual skills are a prerequisite for higher-order learning. Some of its proponents were influenced by the notion of the great Swiss developmental psychologist, Piaget (1960), that all learning is based on a sensorimotor foundation.

Vellutino argued against this kind of analysis, maintaining that the relationship between perceptual and cognitive functioning is probably not sequential, but reciprocal: not only do our concepts develop as a consequence of what we perceive, but what we perceive depends on our existing concepts—this latter point was elaborated in Chapter 2. Also, Vellutino suggested, the perception remediators have misunderstood Piaget on this point—he made it clear that sensory input is understood in the context of established cognitive schemes.

Vellutino concluded that Piaget's theory in fact suggests that remedial activity would be better directed at the acquisition of concepts and relationships that would improve perceptual efficiency, rather than the other way round. However, it seems to me that if the relationship between perception and cognition is truly reciprocal, then it is as valid on theoretical grounds to work from the perceptual as from the conceptual end, although the evidence that perceptual skills training really does promote learning is not strong.

Although this book is mainly about vision, a further brief word is appropriate here about the development of phonological skills, since the optometrist Rosner has addressed himself to this as well as to visual perceptual skills. It was mentioned earlier in the chapter that there is some evidence that poor phonological skills can precede poor reading, and that this can be prevented by appropriate intervention. As far as the experimental evidence is concerned, then, Rosner is perhaps on stronger grounds here than in terms of the visual perceptual aspects of his programme. It is interesting to note, however, the findings of Ellis (1988), which indicated that 'Reading is the pace-maker of. . .phonological processing skills'. His findings on young children suggested that reading appears to promote the development of phonological skills at 5 and 6 years of age, after which they promote one another—again, suggesting a reciprocal relationship between perception and cognition.

In sum, it has to be admitted that the evidence for the effectiveness of perceptual skills training for learning problems is not strong. Vellutino has argued that if a child is having academic difficulties, then remediation should be aimed at that particular academic skill. Many psychologists and teachers would agree with this: if a child cannot read, the appropriate approach is to teach him or her to read, using an individualized programme of instruction that builds on the child's particular strengths. Vellutino believes it sets unnecessary limits to approach the problem from the point of view of the child's deficits. Essentially the same argument can be made in seeking ways to promote the development of children with disabilities (Chapters 7 and 8).

Reading ability and optometric status

It has been suggested for years that there might be a relationship between refractive status and reading ability. It was shown in Chapter 3 that there is a stereotype that adults who wear spectacles are more intelligent, and bright children in cartoons and television advertisements are similarly often portrayed as bespectacled. It seems appropriate to consider in this chapter whether there is any truth at all lying behind the stereotype, and whether there are any implications for the optometrist who deals with children.

A considerable number of studies has been carried out in an effort to determine whether there is, in fact, any relationship between a child's optometric status and reading ability, and reviews of these have been carried out. Some drawbacks of the usual narrative type of review were pointed out by Simons and Gassler (1988), who chose to carry out a meta-analysis of the literature instead. Although this technique is not without its problems, it does enable the results from studies which have looked at similar variables to be combined statistically. This is particularly useful when there is a large number of such studies which do not produce a clear consensus. Of 140 relevant studies identified, Simons and Gassler identified 34 which met their criteria for inclusion in the meta-analysis.

They found that the following were associated with below average reading performance: hyperopia, exophoria at near, vertical phoria, anismetropia and aniseikonia. Myopia and esophoria and exophoria at far were associated with average and above average reading performance. A number of other measures were not associated with reading performance: these were reduced distance acuity, astigmatism, esophoria at near, fusional convergence and divergence, strabismus, nearpoint of convergence and stereopsis.

Hyperopia may cause problems in reading because of the extra accommodative effort needed, producing symptoms such as blurring of print, letters running together and inability to sustain reading. Three possible reasons can be proposed for the association between myopia and average or above average reading ability. Children with myopia are adapted for near tasks, and so may actually find reading easier than other children; their poor distance acuity may cause them to participate less in sporting activities, and spend more time on near activities such as reading; there is also the possibility that reading a great deal causes myopia. Certain binocular problems, such as exophoria at near and vertical phorias, may also be associated with lower reading ability as a result of discomfort which makes reading difficult.

Yet again, there is the problem that the relationships between optometric status and reading ability are correlational, and causality cannot be assumed. Simons and Gassler (1988) make the point that, scientifically speaking, there is no justification for correcting a visual anomaly solely for the purpose of improving reading. However, there are often good optometric reasons for doing so, and individual patients with a high degree of anomaly and eye strain symptoms may well have reading problems as a result.

Conclusion: what should the optometrist be doing?

This chapter may have come across as rather negative in tone, but this is perhaps inevitable given the subject matter. The evidence seems to indicate most strongly that dyslexia is a cognitive developmental problem, and not a visually based disorder. Certainly, visual explanations have little or nothing to say about the spelling problems dyslexics experience. It is, nevertheless, possible that visual problems contribute to learning difficulties in various ways, even if they are not a major cause.

Firstly, there may be conventional optometric problems which make reading uncomfortable, and the correction of these by normal optometric means is obviously desirable: even if a child's dyslexia results from a phonological problem, it will not help if he or she is experiencing eye-strain as a result of hyperopia. The first duty of the optometrist, then, when seeing a child with reading problems, is to carry out a thorough optometric examination and prescribe any necessary correction.

Is the optometrist to offer or recommend any other kind of remediation? On the basis of the available evidence, I believe he or she would be on very shaky ground, and I have serious doubts about the ethics of offering a therapy of unproven effectiveness for monetary gain. However, the parents of dyslexic children are often quite desperate to get help for their children, and may feel neglected by the education system and keen to look elsewhere. They are often very clued-up about the latest therapies which are being promoted, and may come to the optometrist asking for help to implement a particular therapy.

Miles (1988) has considered how the professional is to deal with the situation in which a client asks for a treatment in which the counsellor does not believe (what he calls a 'brussels sprout treatment'). The first requirement of a sceptical counsellor, he says, is to make an honest attempt to evaluate the evidence, and that I have tried to do in this chapter.

Next, he says, it is necessary to weigh up the pros and cons of advising for or against the treatment, considering the potential harm as well as good that might arise in each case. The professional should be frank with the patient about the doubts which exist, but not totally discouraging; the professional's view about the value of the treatment may conceivably be wrong, and in any case the child may benefit from placebo effects. The choice has to lie, ultimately, with the individuals seeking help, but it is only right to point out that they face possible disappointment and a waste of time (and money, if the treatment is expensive).

I outlined earlier my advice with regard to the Irlen treatment: there may be something in it, as yet unproven, but cheap coloured transparent overlays should be as effective as expensive screening and tinted lenses. I am not convinced about the value of eye movement training nor of perceptual skills training. I am also dubious about the reference eye work, but feel it is rather better substantiated than the other treatments; monocular occlusion therapy might be worth trying in the case of a child in whom it has been demonstrated objectively that a stable reference eye has not developed. However, the number of children it might help is small, and patients should be advised about this.

A proviso I would make is that any type of visual treatment should not be seen as a replacement for good teaching assistance, but as an adjunct to it, and co-operation with the child's school should be sought. There is evidence that one-to-one remedial teaching is the best way of making progress when a child experiences reading difficulties (Lundberg, 1985), regardless of the particular theory underlying the teaching; the more individual help the child has, the better the progress.

However, the optometrist need not feel hopeless when it comes to dealing with reading problems in children. He or she can be of help by acting as a counsellor, listening sympathetically, being fully informed about the possibilities, and offering traditional optometric services. The parents of dyslexic children are usually grateful for whatever information they can obtain, even if it is just that their child has normal vision.

References

Abrahamsson M., Sjostrand J. (1986). Impairment of contrast sensitivity function as a measure of disability glare. *Invest. Ophthalmol. Vision Sci.*, **27**, 1131–6.

Adler L., Atwood M. (1987). Poor readers. What do they really see on the page? Unpublished manuscript.

Bishop D. (1987). Unstable vergence control as a cause of specific reading impairment (developmental dyslexia)—a critique. Paper presented to meeting of Academia Rodinensis, Royal Society, London.

Bradley L., Bryant P. (1983). Categorising sounds and learning to read: a causal connection. *Nature*, **301**, 419.

Brown A.M. (1986). Scotopic sensitivity of the 2-month-old human infant. *Vision Res.*, **26**, 707–10.

Chelva E., Collins D.W.K., Levy T.L., McLaren T.L. (1986). Preliminary electrophysiological testing of subjects with prescribed Irlen tinted lenses. Paper presented at Dyslexia Research Foundation Seminar, Perth, W.A., May 1986.

Clayton P. (1987). Scotopic sensitivity. *Optician*, Sept. 25, 22.

Coltheart M. (1980). Analysing reading disorders. Unpublished clinical tests, Bircbeck College, University of London.

Dunlop D.B., Dunlop P., Fenelon B. (1973). Vision laterality analysis in children with reading disability. *Cortex*, **9**, 227.

Ellis A.W. (1983). *Reading, Writing and Dyslexia*. London: Erlbaum.

Ellis N. (1988). The development of literacy and short-term memory. In *Practical Aspects of Memory II* (Gruneberg M.M., Morris P.E., Sykes R.N., eds). Chichester: Wiley.

Fowler M.S., Riddell P.M., Stein J.F. (1988). The effect of varying vergence speed and target size on the amplitude of vergence eye movements. *Br. Orthoptic J.*, **45**, 49–55.

Frith U. (1981). Experimental approaches to developmental dyslexia: an introduction. *Psychol. Res.*, **43**, 97–109.

Frostig M. (1961). *The Marianne Frostig Developmental Test of Visual Perception*. Palo Alto, California: Consulting Psychology Press.

Gregg P.J. (1988). Dyslexia and tinted lenses. A small research project. *Optician*, Jan. 29, 17–20.

Hammill D.D., Larsen S.C., Parker R. et al. (1974). Perceptual and conceptual correlates of reading. Unpublished manuscript, 1505 Sunny Vale, Austin, Texas.

Hartje W. (1972). Reading disturbances in the presence of oculomotor disorders. *Eur. Neurol.*, **7**, 249–64.

Herrin S. (1985). Is there hope for vision training? *Rev. Optom.*, May, 23–28.

Howell E., Stanley G. (1988). Colour and learning disability. *Clin. Exp. Optom.*, **71**, 66–71.

Irlen H. (1983). Successful treatment of learning disabilities. Paper presented to American Psychological Association, Aug. 1983.

Larsen S.C., Hammill D.D. (1975). The relationship of selected visual-perceptual abilities to school learning. *J. Special Ed.*, **9**, 281–91.

Lundberg I. (1985). Longitudinal studies of reading and reading disability in Sweden. In *Reading Research: Advances in Theory and Practice* vol.4 (Mackinnon G.E., Waller T.G., eds). London: Academic Press, pp. 65–105.

Marshall J.C. (1984). Toward a rational taxonomy of the developmental dyslexias. In *Dyslexia: A Global Issue* (Malatesha R.N., Whitaker H.A., eds). The Hague: Martinus Nijhoff.

Masters M.C. (1988). Orthoptic management of visual dyslexia. *Br. Orthoptic J.*, **45**, 40–8.

Miles T.R. (1987). *Understanding Dyslexia*. Bath: Better Books.

Miles T.R. (1988). Counselling in dyslexia. *Counselling Psychol. Q.*, **1**, 97–107.

Millodot M. (1986). *Dictionary of Optometry*. London: Butterworths.

Morton J. (1969). Interaction of information in word recognition. *Psychol. Rev.*, **76**, 165–78.

Murphy C.N. Diagnosis and remediation for scotopic sensitivity syndrome. Unpublished manuscript.

Newman S. (1987). The Dunlop test, reading and spelling. Paper presented to meeting of Academia Rodinensis, Royal Society, London.

Ogle K. (1962). The optical space sense. In *The Eye* vol. IV (Darson H., ed.). New York: Academic Press.

Orton S.T. (1937). *Reading, Writing and Speech Problems in Children*. London: Chapman & Hall.

Pavlidis G. (1981). Sequencing eye movements and the early objective diagnosis of dyslexia. In *Dyslexia Research and its Applications to Education* (Pavlidis G., Miles T., eds). London: Wiley.

Pavlidis G. (1983). The 'dyslexia syndrome' and its objective diagnosis by erratic eye movements. In: *Eye Movements in Reading: Perceptual and Language Processes* (Rayner K., ed.). New York: Academic.

Piaget J. (1960). Développement et apprentissage perceptis. In *Proceedings of the 16th International Congress of Psychology*. Bonn, pp. 223–225.

Pirozzolo F. J. (1983). Eye movements and reading disability. In *Eye Movements in Reading: Perceptual and Language Processes* (Rayner K., ed.). New York: Academic Press.

Pollatsek A. (1983). What can eye movements tell us about dyslexia? In *Eye Movements in Reading: Perceptual and Language Processes* (Rayner K., ed.). New York: Academic Press.

Porac C., Coren S. (1978). *Am. J. Optom. Physiol. Opt.*, **55**, 208.

Raymond J.E., Ogden N. A., Fagan J.E., Kaplan B.J. (1988). Fixational instability and saccadic eye movements of dyslexic children with subtle cerebellar dysfunction. *Am. J. Optom. Physiol. Opt.*, **65**, 174–81.

Reeves B. (1988). Reading through rose-tinted spectacles. *Optician*, Jan. 29, 21–6.

Richardson A.S. (1988). The utilisation of coloured filters to reduce scotopic sensitivity. Undergraduate project, Dept. of Psychology, University College of Wales, Swansea.

Riddell P.M., Stein J.F., Fowler M.S. (1987). A comparison of sighting dominance and the reference eye in reading disabled children. *Br. Orthoptic J.*, **44**, 64–9.

Robinson G.L., Miles J. (1987). The use of coloured overlays to improve visual processing—a preliminary survey. *Except. Child*, **34**, 65–70.

Rosner J. (1979). *Helping Children Overcome Learning Difficulties*. New York: Walker Educational Books.

Rosner J., Rosner J. (1986). The clinical management of perceptual skills disorders in a primary care practice. *J. Am. Optom. Assoc.*, **57**, 56–9.

Rosner J., Rosner J. (1987). The Irlen treatment: a review of the literature. *Optician*, Sept. 25, 26–33.

Sabatino D.A., Abbott J.C., Becker J.T. (1974). What does the Frostig DTVP measure? *Except. Child*, **40**, 453–4.

Saint-John L.M. (1986). The effect of coloured transparencies on the reading performance of specifically reading disabled children. Tasmanian State Institute of Technology, B.Ed. project.

Shute R. (1991). Treating dyslexia with tinted lenses: a review of the evidence. *Res. Ed.* (in press).

Shute R., Paton D. (1990). Childhood illness: the child as helper. In *Children Helping Children* (Foot H., Morgan M., Shute R., eds). Chichester: J. Wiley.

Simons H.D., Gassler P.A. (1988). Vision anomalies and reading skills: a meta-analysis of the literature. *Am. J. Optom. Physiol. Opt.*, **11**, 893–904.

Snowling M. (1987). *Dyslexia. A Cognitive Developmental Perspective.* Oxford: Blackwell.

Stanley P.M. Study of scotopic sensitivity: benefits from photopic transmittent lenses. Unpublished manuscript.

Stanley G., Smith G.A., Howell E.A. (1983). Eye movements and sequential tracking in dyslexic and control children. *Br. J. Psychol.*, **74**, 181–7.

Stein J.F., Fowler M.S. (1985). Effects of monocular occlusion on visuomotor perception and reading in dyslexic children. *Lancet*, **ii**, 69–73.

Stein J. (1987). Reply to Bishop. Meeting of *Academia Rodensis*. Royal Society, London.

Stein J., Riddell P.M., Fowler M.S. (1987). Fine binocular control in dyslexic children. *Eye*, **1**, 433–8.

Vellutino F.R. (1987). Dyslexia. *Sci. Am.*, **256**, 34–41.

Vellutino F.R., Steger B.M., Moyer B. et al. (1977). Has the perceptual deficit hypothesis led us astray? *J. Learning Disabilities*, **10**, 375–85.

Wilkins A. (1990). Paper presented to meeting of Academia Rodinensis, Royal Society, London.

Winter S. (1986). Irlen lenses. An appraisal. Unpublished manuscript.

World Federation of Neurology (1968). Cited by Critchley (1970). *The Dyslexic Child*. London: Heinemann Medical Books.

Chapter 7

Patients with special needs

Introduction

From time to time, any optometrist will come across patients with special needs which stem from physical or intellectual impairments, or from a combination of problems. While the vision care of such patients can sometimes be time-consuming and needs special skills, it is becoming increasingly feasible: even those with severe communication problems are now testable, largely as a result of the availability of techniques first developed within the context of infant vision testing. Patients with special needs can benefit enormously from proper vision care, but this is often not provided.

Optometrists working within hospitals are particularly likely to come across such patients, and some in private practice may wish to consider specializing, if only partially, in providing care for patients with special needs. This can be done by making arrangements with institutions such as special schools, day care centres and hospitals. Examples of optometrists who have adopted this practice are Puzio (1984) in the USA, who provides vision care for autistic children and adults with intellectual impairment, and Davies (personal communication), who provides vision care for patients in a hospital stroke unit in South Wales.

Attitudes towards those with special needs are currently undergoing change, not least as a result of pressure from such people themselves. There has been a great deal of discussion about appropriate terminology and the meanings of such words as 'disability' and 'handicap'. With reference to low vision, Lovie-Kitchin and Bowman (1985) have made a distinction between impairment, disability and handicap: an impairment is a limitation of function, a disability a limitation of ability to perform certain tasks, and a handicap is the disadvantage a person experiences because of a disability.

Others have discussed the use of the term 'disability', advocating a move away from an individual definition to a sociopolitical definition: a disability is not something that resides in the individuals concerned, but within society's attitudes towards them. On this view, for example, those who use a wheelchair are not inherently disabled, but may be disabled if inadequate provision of ramps prevents them from accessing places others take for granted (Dever, 1988). This could be considered an example of handicap, rather than disability, using the definitions given above. Whichever terminology is preferred, the intention is the same—to remove the problem as an inherent aspect of the individual into the environment, whether this be the physical circumstances in which the person has to operate or the social environment with its attitudes towards people with special needs. The failure to provide vision care for people with special needs is adding to the disability (or handicap) that they experience; within the limits of available techniques, vision care should be as accessible to those with special needs as to the rest of the community. Indeed, making the most of their vision may be even more vital for those who must face life with additional physical and/or intellectual problems.

Those promoting the sociopolitical view of disability also argue against the use of a linguistic style which defines individuals in terms of their conditions. Referring to someone as 'a disabled person' or 'a diabetic', for example, suggests that he or she is a complaint with a person attached, rather than a person who happens to have a particular condition. It is proposed that such phrases should be replaced by those which append the condition to the person, for example, 'a person with a disability' or 'a person with diabetes'. In writing this book I have attempted in the main to avoid the prejudicial language just described, although I confess to resorting to it occasionally for the sake of readability. Other common phrases have also come under attack: a person may not necessarily be 'suffering from' a condition, for example, but be well adjusted to it, while others do not see themselves as 'confined' to wheelchairs, but are appreciative of the mobility they afford.

In dealing with the parents of children with disabilities, the optometrist needs to be understanding about the emotional aspects of the situation. Particularly in the early days after the birth, the parents may be mourning the loss of the perfect child they expected but did not have. They may be angry, and express this towards medical and other workers involved with the baby (Weinmann, 1987). Later they may become depressed, before accepting the situation, but some remain embarrassed by the child's condition and tend to withdraw socially. In any case, these parents are likely to be under continuing stress as a result of the extra time and attention the child needs. They are often keen to obtain as much information as possible about the child's abilities and prognosis, so it is important to be as informative as possible (bearing in mind the guidelines on information-giving outlined in Chapter 4), but neither dashing hopes insensitively nor raising false ones. Ways of avoiding the development of an adversarial relationship with the parents of disabled children were discussed in Chapter 5.

Children with physical impairments become aware of them around the age of school entry, and may accept the situation reasonably well at first. However, as the child matures, and particularly in adolescence, there may be stronger emotional reactions, and possibly denial of the difficulties, until acceptance is again reached. More is said about the process of denial and how the practitioner should handle it in the final chapter, with reference to visual loss.

People do not behave in the same way towards those with disabilities as to the able-bodied. As discussed elsewhere, emotional responses are expressed non-verbally; patterns of eye contact, smiling and proximity change when people interact with the disabled, and those with disabilities are sensitive to this (Comer and Piliavin, 1972). These non-verbal cues to discomfort are not present in people who are used to interacting with people with disabilities. The optometrist who feels uneasy at the prospect of meeting such patients can take heart from the fact that this may well improve with experience, and those with disabilities are often very good at dealing with other people's reactions and discomfort (an exception is the first patient group to be considered, those with intellectual impairments, whose condition restricts the degree of insight they have into the feelings of other people).

The patient with intellectual impairment

People with intellectual impairments have in the past been referred to by a number of terms which are now considered to be stigmatizing, including 'subnormal' and 'mentally handicapped'. Increasingly, they are referred to as 'people with learning difficulties', since these lie at the core of their problems. Even this term can cause confusion, however, especially in a book such as this which also considers specific learning problems such as dyslexia, and this is why, in consultation with Dever (personal communication) I have chosen the term 'intellectual impairment'.

This can result from chromosomal abnormality (such as Down's syndrome), trauma, hypoxia, prenatal infection, prematurity, metabolic disease, toxins and neurological disease. However, in about half of cases the cause is unknown. The learning problems may stem from a short attention span or poor short-term memory, but the extent of the difficulty varies enormously. It was fashionable, at one time, to categorize people with intellectual impairments on the basis of IQ scores: in comparison with the population average of 100, those with an IQ of 70 or less were considered to have an intellectual impairment, and terms such as 'idiot' and 'moron' were used to indicate particular levels of IQ. The fact that such words have become converted into terms of abuse says something about the attitudes of society towards intellectual impairment. Nowadays, there is a move away from categorization towards considering the special needs of each child, based not simply on an IQ score but on the total circumstances of the child, and naturalistic observations supplement formal tests (Smith and Cowie, 1988).

Those with intellectual impairment are at high risk of ocular anomaly, those with the severest intellectual impairment are also most likely to have a high degree of visual difficulty (Warburg, 1970, 1982). Woodruff (1977) found visual anomalies in two-thirds of a sample of Canadian children with intellectual impairment living in the community, and in a Danish study 5% of children with intellectual impairment had a visual acuity of less than 6/60, compared with a fraction of 1% in the rest of the child population (Warburg, 1982). In 228 institutionalized adults, of whom nearly a quarter had Down's syndrome, Jacobson (1988) found that more than half had one or more ocular disorders, a quarter having a considerable visual handicap; in some cases, this was unknown before her study.

Jacobson's study is indicative of the kinds of visual anomalies to be expected. She found a high incidence of optic atrophy, high myopia, cataract, retinal disease and keratoconus. Many had considerable anisometropia or only one good eye (10% had anisometropia of more than two dioptres, which is 10 times the normal rate). Considering the better eye, 23% had considerable refractive error, compared with about 12% of the general population.

Efforts to provide vision care for this patient group, particularly those who are institutionalized, may meet with scepticism, not least among the medical profession. There are often doubts as to whether the effort put in will be worth it in terms of improving the lives of these people who, it is often thought, are unlikely to use any spectacles anyway. One indication of the present state of vision care provision for patients with intellectual impairments is the fact that Jacobson (1988) could find no previous literature on intraocular surgery for these patients. Another is that a sample of London ophthalmologists reported that they felt unable to accept any more patients with intellectual impairments for routine services (Harries, 1989).

Those who lobby for better provision would argue that they have as much right to good vision as those in the general population. In addition, there are reports of the value of providing vision care for even the most severely affected. In Jacobson's (1988) study, adults in an institution were followed up 6–12 months after the prescription of refractive corrections. Those with myopia tolerated their spectacles well, were more mobile, could climb stairs and showed a greater interest in their surroundings. Bifocals for presbyopia were also well tolerated, the wearers took a more active part in close work and were responding well to training in daily activities. These results must be interpreted somewhat cautiously, as the precise ways in which these behaviour changes were measured is not reported, and it is possible that the nursing staff changed their own behaviours and assessments of the patients as a result of the study. However, it was reported that those with hypermetropia did not respond so favourably to their spectacles, and this may be an indication that the changes in behaviour noted in the other spectacle wearers were genuinely due to improved vision. This study confirms earlier reports (Warburg, 1964, 1970) that many people with intellectual impairments will use spectacles if they are prescribed. Jacobson also reported that intraocular surgery was carried out on 14 patients, with subsequent improvement in vision in 8, and with no complications (those who did not show improved vision were found to have optic atrophy or retinal damage).

Down's syndrome is the commonest cause of intellectual impairment, affecting around 1 baby in 500, and therefore warrants particular consideration. A child with Down's syndrome may not be noticeably different in development from other children at first, but is likely to begin to fall behind by the end of the first year (Lewis, 1987). However, there is evidence that early intervention, before 6 months, promotes good development. At this stage, the parents may still be struggling to come to terms with their child's condition. Like any other health care worker, the optometrist needs to be aware of this, and to be able to provide accurate information sensitively to parents about the child's vision. Assuming the child's vision is in the normal range for his or her age, it may be particularly reassuring for parents to be told this.

The baby and young child with Down's seem to take longer to process information than other children: they may need to look and listen to stimuli for longer in order to recognize them, and are slower to smile or laugh. It is important, therefore, during testing, to give them enough time to respond. They may also forget skills they have demonstrated previously, and so may be erratic during assessment. It may be worthwhile, therefore, to see a child with Down's more frequently than usual, particularly if his or her visual performance seems low.

It is now known that many children with Down's are more capable than previously thought; many learn to read, pass examinations and find employment. However, they are likely to experience age-related visual problems earlier than the rest of the population (Jacobson, 1988). It is particularly vital, therefore, that their vision is monitored to enable them to keep up early progress: one young man of 14 attended Cardiff's Low Vision Clinic because of developing cataracts, and was able to make use of a magnifier to keep up his reading at school.

It is generally assumed, when testing children, that their accommodation will be good. However, this may not be the case in Down's syndrome. Meades et al. (1990), using dynamic retinoscopy, found reduced accommodative capacity in children with Down's. The implication of this is that some of the children may require reading aids, either in the form of bifocals or separate reading glasses.

Many people with an intellectual impairment display unusual social behaviours, as their learning problems are general ones, extending to the learning of socially acceptable behaviours. Some are very socially unresponsive, not making eye contact or communicating verbally. On the other hand, there are those who speak loudly, make statements which appear irrelevant to the situation or try to hug people they don't know well! People who are not used to this tend to feel uncomfortable about it, and this may include other patients in the waiting room. An optometrist providing vision care for these patients in the high street must make an individual decision, based on personal moral values, about whether or not to consider the feelings of other patients who may have difficulty in dealing with this situation, by booking in such patients at quiet times (perhaps at the end of a morning or afternoon). The alternative, which those who champion the rights of the disabled would argue, is to treat all patients on an equal footing and regard any 'regular' patients who find difficulty with this as the ones with the problem (bearing in mind the sociopolitical definition of disability referred to earlier, by which disability lies in the attitudes of society, not in the individual concerned).

While any patient may be apprehensive about vision testing, some patients with intellectual impairments may be frankly afraid: they may fear new people and situations in general, or they may have had unpleasant medical experiences in the past. It is the practice both in the Cardiff Visual Assessment Unit and in Puzio's work with autistic patients not to wear a white coat, which may be associated with previous medical experiences. In Cardiff Visual Assessment Unit we find that some patients from institutions are very apologetic, saying they are sorry for events for which they have no responsibility, such as the optometrist tripping over or dropping something. It is not clear whether they have a history of being blamed when things go wrong or whether they have intellectual difficulty with attributing causality to events. Whatever the reason, plenty of reassurance and the presence of a relative or other carer during testing are very important.

Some patients may be quite capable of understanding what is happening during vision testing if simple explanations are given, and be able to co-operate with the usual procedures. Some are perfectly able to respond to a Snellen chart or to children's tests such as the Sheridan-Gardiner.

For others, acuity cards provide a useful alternative. Duckman and Selenow (1983) examined the proposition that forced choice preferential looking (the acuity card procedure) will remain suitable at a later age than usual for children who are developmentally delayed, and obtained clear preferential looking responses in 11 of 12 children tested, aged between 6 months and 3½ years.

Hertz (1987) tested Down's syndrome children with acuity cards and found results which compared well with those obtained using the Østerberg picture chart. The majority of children responded well, by speech, gesture or fixation, but they became frustrated near threshold, and a third alternative, 'no stripes', had to be given to them. Number of presentations had to be kept to a minimum. She also used the acuity cards to test intellectually impaired children with cerebral palsy: again, useful information was obtained, although results were more variable in this group. She noted that carers report that these children appear to see better on some days than others, and this may have contributed to the variability. Hertz (1988) also examined the reliability of testing children with cerebral palsy plus severe intellectual impairment, and found reliable measurements in those with acuity better than 2/60.

Chandna et al. (1989) examined the feasibility of carrying out preferential looking with adults with intellectual impairments. They found a good correlation with Snellen acuity, the vast majority of measurements using the two methods being within 0.5 octave of one another. It was not, however, possible to measure acuity in all patients, and a few of the most profoundly impaired could not even be tested using the Catford drum. Some patients became anxious if the tester disappeared behind the cards (reminiscent of the difficulty infants have in understanding objects which disappear), and in these cases the tester remained in view.

Experience in the Cardiff Visual Assessment Unit is in accordance with that of other workers, who have noted the short attention span of those with intellectual impairments, and the need to streamline procedures. A new set of acuity cards, the Cardiff Acuity Cards, using more interesting targets than stripes, is currently under development, with the aim of improving attention to testing (Woodhouse, personal communication).

Jacobson (1988) and Shentall and Hosking (1986) have found that some patients respond better to non-symbolic tests (such as being able to see the cake decorations hundreds-of-thousands, indicating a visual acuity of at least 6/60) than to symbolic tests, such as the Østerberg picture chart.

A combined test of acuity and visual form perception for use with children with visual and/or intellectual impairments has been developed by Lindstedt (1986). The test consists of a set of playing cards, the BUST-LH cards, which display symbols of different sizes. The theoretical background of the test is based on an analysis of the complex procedures and skills necessary in most other available vision tests, including attentiveness, memory and ability to general-ize. The tester can use the cards flexibly, playing games with the patient, to gain an indication of functional acuity.

The various techniques and findings discussed above indicate the need for and feasibility of providing vision care for the majority of children and adults with intellectual impairments. If they are tested at an early age, then any necessary interventions can be carried out to minimize permanent visual impairment and aid general develop-ment. However, it is never too late to provide vision care: if, as findings suggest, patients become more mobile and more able to carry out everyday activities, then carers such as family and nursing staff will be freed from some of the mundane tasks of helping with routine activities such as feeding and helping to negotiate stairs, and concentrate instead on working on higher level activities with the patients. Improved vision also means that those who move out of institutions into the community will have a better chance of being able to cope.

The patient with a hearing impairment

The title I have given this section takes account of the discussion on terminology: these patients are people who happen to have a hearing difficulty, rather than people who are defined by deafness. However, repeatedly using this phrase makes for clumsy writing, and I have never come across the alternative term 'people with deafness'. Since those with severe hearing impairments refer to themselves as 'the deaf' and 'deaf people', I have considered it acceptable to use these terms occasionally for the sake of readability.

It is important that the visual needs of those with hearing impairments are met. Those who have a loss in the auditory modality will be particularly dependent on vision, for signing, lipreading and a whole range of other visual cues as to what is occurring in their environment.

Sometimes, especially if the hearing loss is profound, the optometrist will have been made aware of this from the outset, and will be conscious of the possibility of deafness in association with certain visual defects, such as retinitis pigmentosa. In other cases, though, it may only become apparent during the consultation that the patient has a hearing problem. Indicative behaviours by the patient include: asking for questions to be repeated; giving answers that do not make sense; misinterpreting instructions; cupping a hand behind the ear; leaning forward; staring at the optometrist's lips; speaking loudly. Given such indications, Karp (1984) advises against asking a patient 'How is your hearing?', as the reply is often that it is fine. Instead, she suggests asking 'Has your hearing loss reached a handicapping level?', and referring a patient who wishes it for medical attention.

The most profound effect of congenital deafness is in the area of language acquisition, which is a slow, painstaking process. Although some deaf people have excellent communication skills, the majority have serious language impairment. In terms of speech, even teachers of the deaf have difficulty in understanding three-quarters of their pupils with a hearing loss of over 90 dB (Conrad, 1981). Communication is therefore the basic problem which the optometrist faces with such a patient, especially as he or she is unlikely to be familiar with any signing system, such as Makaton, which the patient may use.

The optometrist needs information about the particular method of communication used by the patient, and an interpreter, such as a relative, is invaluable if the patient uses a signing system. Verma (1988) suggests that the optometrist keeps an electronic amplifying device, or even a stethoscope, available, as these may aid communication with some patients who are hard-of-hearing. Some people who have experienced a gradual hearing loss may have come to rely on lipreading without consciously realizing it. It is important to face patients who lipread and articulate clearly, but it is not necessary (and insulting) to indulge in exaggerated pantomime. Vision of at least 5/80 is required for lipreading (Karp, 1984), and this is an important factor to consider if the patient has low vision as well as a hearing loss. It must also be borne in mind that patients will be unable to lipread when being tested in the dark, or when the optometrist is reaching across for lenses or holding a retinoscope in front of the face. Some ingenuity may also be needed to overcome problems during subjective testing as a result of lenses causing blurred vision. Being deprived of verbal aspects of communication, including such cues as tone of voice, a deaf person may be particularly sensitive to non-verbal behaviour, and the optometrist therefore needs to be especially aware of this. In particular, although speaking more loudly than usual may be helpful, the practitioner should not shout, as the accompanying non-verbal signals may unintentionally convey anger.

Several studies have suggested that deaf children have a higher than average risk of ocular problems (e.g. Suchman 1968). It is therefore especially important that they are screened to enable any visual problems to be detected and remediated at an early age, otherwise the child will be at a double sensory disadvantage which has profound developmental implications. The types of visual problem to be anticipated are related to the cause of deafness. According to Woodruff's (1986) Canadian study, fewest visual anomalies are associated with inherited deafness, while congenital rubella is associated with a wide range (there appears to be a significant effect on corneal curvature, resulting in a broad spectrum of spherical refractive errors). Higher rates of strabismus and amblyopia occur with neonatal sepsis and rhesus incompatibility. These two conditions are also respectively associated with hyperopia and myopia, while children whose deafness resulted from meningitis are more likely to be hyperopic.

While children and younger people with hearing impairments are a very important patient group, it is the case that most people with hearing impairments are over the age of 65 (Karp, 1984).

Many older patients will have a hearing loss which is only marginal, but Rabbitt (1988) has reported that even this can can have adverse social effects: not only are they likely to mishear what is said, but listening is more effortful, thus making remembering what has been said more difficult. He points out that 'even slightly deaf elderly people may seem more stupid than they really are, and project quite unjust images of their true capabilities'. He calls for more humane and tolerant judgements. On the practical side, the comments above about articulating clearly and permitting lipreading are equally applicable to the slightly deaf. In addition, there should be no interfering background noise, such as music. Since remembering what has been said may be more difficult for the hearing–impaired, in addition to the problems which all patients can have in remembering information and advice (Chapter 4), it seems especially advisable to provide written reminders for such patients. Some patients with more profound hearing loss may in any case communicate by means of written notes, which can serve a dual purpose as take-home reminders.

Type of hearing aid used is a consideration when prescribing spectacles or low vision aids, and interprofessional contact with the audiologist is needed when a patient has both low vision and a hearing impairment. For example, if a person's vision is too poor for adequate orientation and mobility, some compensation can be achieved by providing hearing aids which balance hearing in the two ears [see Karp (1984) for further discussion].

The patient with multiple impairments

Patients with multiple impairments (often referred to as multiply

handicapped) present perhaps the greatest challenge to the optometrist. Such patients may have some or all of the following
problems: intellectual impairment, mobility problems, co-
ordination problems, communication difficulties, hearing impairment, low vision, behavioural problems and perhaps additional
health problems. A whole host of different circumstances may give
rise to these multiple problems, including inherited conditions,
prenatal or perinatal problems (such as maternal rubella or
prematurity) and later illness or accident.

Such people are at higher than average risk of visual problems,
but Hill (1987) has pointed out that many optometrists and
ophthalmologists have been frustrated by the fact that these patients
do not respond to standard testing procedures, and persons with
severe disabilities are often excluded from vision screening programmes (Cress et al., 1981). They may also be denied treatment,
such as surgery and corrective lenses (Hill, 1987). Orel-Bixler et al.
(1989) examined 59 patients between the ages of 3 and 33 years;
they found significant refractive error in 73%, strabismus in 71%,
and nystagmus in 36%. Only 37% with significant refractive error
were wearing their proper correction, and uncorrected refractive
errors from -10 to $+20D$ were found.

As in the case of intellectual impairment, new methods enable
patients with multiple difficulties to be examined, and I and my
colleagues in the Visual Assessment Unit at Cardiff would certainly
agree with Hill's sentiment that nobody should be regarded as
untestable, regardless of age or the multiplicity of the problems.

Many multiply impaired infants are visually unresponsive. Harrison (1985) has argued for early visual assessment as part of the
process of avoiding the establishment of 'disabled' patterns and
attitudes.

Rogow et al. (1984) have made a similar point, arguing that when
the major clinical signs are lack of fixation and tracking, the term
'blind' should not be used, as attempts will then not be made to
stimulate the child visually (this is also discussed in Chapter 8). They
point out that children with central nervous system damage may not
show the usual visual orienting responses; even those with a viable
visual system may have difficulty with perceiving, interpreting or
acting upon visual stimuli, and visual behaviour may never develop.
However, they claim that with good interprofessional co-operation,
including 'prompt and careful attention from the optometrical and
medical professions. . .severe and profound retardation and visual
avoidance may be prevented in most of these children', who must
be taught to look.

Information in advance from carers is very helpful for planning
the kinds of provisions for vision testing that will need to be made.
The optometrist needs to be aware of any special communication

system which the patient uses, such as gestures. Unwarranted assumptions about intellectual impairment should not be made, as someone with severe physical and communication difficulties may nevertheless be of average or high intelligence. As with all patients with special needs, the optometrist should avoid the 'does he take sugar?' syndrome, and address the patient directly, even if an accompanying person has to interpret.

Orel-Bixler and associates (1989) have discussed ways of measuring the vision of multiply impaired patients. Using a spatial frequency sweep visually evoked potential technique they were able to measure binocular acuities in 95% of patients, and in 70% using acuity cards. Patients' responses to visual corrections are being followed up.

Successful use of acuity cards with children with cerebral palsy has been reported by Hertz and Rosenberg (1988). Although the most severely affected children had greater test–retest variabilities, the majority showed an acceptable agreement.

Experience with multiply impaired patients in the Cardiff Visual Assessment Unit has shown that oculomotor problems can cause difficulty with acuity card testing: if strabismus is present, or there is difficulty in controlling eye movements, it is not always easy to determine where the patient is looking. A simple arrangement of two light-bulbs spaced about 35 cm apart, which can be switched on and off alternately (known as the Leat lights after Dr Sue Leat who devised them) is helpful. This simple arrangement enables the tester to determine whether the patient can reliably move the eyes from one target to another, and to determine any idiosyncrasy which the patient has; for example, some severely affected patients require a considerable time, perhaps as long as 10 s, to change fixation. This knowledge can then be applied to the acuity cards.

It is important to communicate optometric findings to others involved with patients, such as parents, general practitioners, teachers and special needs advisers. The information should be couched in a useful, practical form. A case which illustrates the kind of advice that can be given is that of a young man with intellectual and hearing impairments, low visual acuity and cataracts; he was working with a computer and, following assessment, we advised his teacher to use large, high-contrast targets, with the contrast of the screen turned up to maximum, and to ensure that sunlight did not fall on the screen.

In Cardiff, we see adults who have hitherto had little vision care, reflecting Hill's experience in Canada. For example, one man was brought for his first vision test in his 30s. He had cerebral palsy, used a wheelchair, and had little ability to communicate. Although his mother and 10 siblings had high myopia, no one had ever suggested a test until their attention was drawn to the existence of our clinic. Not surprisingly, ne turned out to require a high minus correction, which was prescribed in two stages. His mother reported that he subsequently showed a greater interest in looking out of the window and in people entering the room. Hopefully, a greater involvement by optometrists with young children with multiple impairments will help to prevent them from becoming the neglected adults of tomorrow.

The adult who has had a stroke or head injury

Optometrists need to be knowledgeable about brain injury, especially stroke, since Cockburn (1983) reported that more than 12% of patients over 50 years of age presenting at an optometric practice had signs or symptoms of completed or impending stroke (and the optometrist has a vital preventive role to play here).

Two people per 1000 of the population suffer a severe cerebrovascular accident (CVA, or stroke) annually (Newcombe, 1985), and this proportion is likely to increase as a result of demographic changes, that is, an increasing proportion of elderly in the population. Of those admitted to hospital (in the UK, less than half the total), three-quarters survive 6 months or longer. Many are left with severe physical, cognitive and emotional problems.

The effects of a CVA will be determined largely by the locus and extent of the damage, and in addition the patient frequently becomes depressed. There may be paresis on the side of the body contralateral to the injury. Around a third to a half of stroke survivors have persistent language impairment (dysphasia), usually associated with left hemisphere damage, although more subtle types of language impairment (such as inability to use paralinguistic features—see Chapter 4) can result from right hemisphere damage. Right hemisphere damage can also lead to visual problems which result not from field losses as such, but from impairment of the higher processing of visual information. There may be a lack of attention to one side of space (unilateral visual neglect); whereas someone with a field defect can compensate to some extent by head movements, the person with neglect does not generally recognize or may even deny the problem, happily leaving his face half-shaved or half a meal unfinished on one side of the plate. Testing for such higher-order visual problems is usually the province of the clinical psychologist, and interprofessional communication is invaluable for the management of such patients.

The other major cause of severe brain damage is closed head injury, such as caused by road traffic accidents, assaults and falls. This tends to result in diffuse neural degeneration, which leaves many with major disabilities, including deficits in memory, attention and intellect as well as emotional disturbances. Sometimes the injury will have extended to the eyes and surrounding area. When a head injury is caused by a penetrating missile, such as a bullet, the pattern of deficit tends to reflect the location of injury, as with CVA.

Sadly, as noted by Newcombe (1985), 'technical advances in neurosurgical care to save life have not always been paralleled by facilities that make the quality of that life tolerable for patient and relatives'. Attempts at rehabilitation have often met with scepticism [e.g. Miller (1984) with regard to dysphasia], but new impetus and a new respectability have been given to rehabilitation because of new insights gained within the realms of clinical neuropsychology and cognitive psychology (Newcombe, 1985; Wilson, 1989).

Clearly, the measurement of visual capacity should form an integral part of the assessment of the brain-injured, as it will influence most other areas of functioning: as noted by Nooney (1986), 'visual rehabilitaton is often one of the first steps in total rehabilitation'. An obvious example is that attempts to remediate lost literacy skills (Shute and Curtis, 1989) will fail if the individual cannot see the page clearly because of the lack of an appropriate prescription for the correction of refractive error. Another example is provided by Freeman and Rudge (1988), who point out that reduced stereopsis may adversely affect the results of tests of motor ability. Other important visual problems often resulting from brain injury include hemianopia and, as mentioned above, visual neglect; these are not always easy to test for nor to distinguish, and yet have profound implications for rehabilitation (e.g. Nooney, 1986; Sunderland et al., 1987; Wade et al., 1988).

Other visual problems which may occur after brain injury include reduced acuity, diplopia, oculomotor nerve palsies, strabismus, reduced convergence and nystagmus (Freeman and Rudge, 1988). There may also be pre-existing conditions, such as diabetic retinopathy, cataract, refractive error and presbyopia, which may or may not have been assessed or treated before the brain injury occurred. However, there is little literature on the implications of brain damage for routine optometric procedures.

Any kind of assessment of a patient with dysphasia is very difficult, and optometric assessment is no exception, since communication between patient and optometrist is a vital part of the testing procedure. Problems may be expressive or receptive in nature, that is, the production of speech or its understanding may be more affected, and there may be corresponding problems with the written word—writing or reading problems. The previous chapter, on reading difficulties in children, outlined current theory about reading processes, and an understanding of this will help to cast light on the kinds of problems experienced by people with certain brain injuries. Some patients have relatively few problems, such as occasional word-finding difficulties, while others may be severely affected all round (globally dysphasic, or aphasic). The presence of a family member or a speech therapist's report is invaluable in preparing to meet the problems of individuals. Some, for example, prefer to write rather than speak, or use sign language or some kind of letter chart; the presence of an interpreter is vital in such cases. Some patients use 'yes' and 'no' inappropriately, and if the optometrist does not know this it can cause considerable confusion. Others with speech problems can give 'yes' and 'no' answers if questions are suitably framed.

Again, as with all patients with special needs, the patient should be addressed personally, and not talked about to carers as if he or she were not present. Many brain-injured patients who cannot speak can nevertheless understand most or all of what is said. Patience must be exercised with those whose speech is hesitant because of word-finding or articulation difficulties.

Acuity may be impaired as a direct result of head trauma, especially where intracranial pressure causes damage to the visual pathways. Testing acuity with a Snellen chart may not be possible for a number of reasons. Patients may be unable to recognize letters, or to articulate their names; there may be more unusual problems such as the inability to deal with upper–case letters or certain letters of the alphabet. Tests such as the Sheridan-Gardiner or Illiterate 'E' may be appropriate for some dysphasics, but not all, since some have impaired matching ability (Sheridan-Gardiner or Cambridge acuity test) while others have problems with orientation (Illiterate 'E'). Visual neglect may affect the tests, also, as the patient will fail to attend to one side of the presented targets.

As with the other patient groups discussed in this chapter, acuity cards can provide a useful means of measuring the acuity of patients with communication problems. Although their use with brain-injured adults has yet to be formally assessed, there are anecdotal reports of its use [for example, Price (1986) reported to Freeman and Rudge (1988)] and they have proved useful with such patients in Cardiff's Visual Assessment Unit. The presence of visual neglect would be expected to affect the use of acuity cards, and if this is thought to be a problem, turning the cards vertically may help.

As mentioned earlier, problems with binocular function frequently follow brain damage (e.g. Tyerman, 1989) but are rarely assessed (Gianutsos and Matheson, 1987). Two non-verbal clinical tests for stereopsis, the Lang and the Frisby, may prove useful with those with communication problems, as they are with older infants (Broadbent and Westall, 1989).

Visual fields should always be tested in patients with brain injury, as field losses frequently occur. They are usually cortical, or at least post-chiasmic, and therefore homonymous, although there may be losses from other causes such as glaucoma. Gianutsos and Matheson (1987) regard testing by confrontation as unsuitable for the brain-injured, as many cases of field loss may be missed. They recommend thorough perimetric examination, preferably using a forced-choice mode rather than a kinetic mode, but not every optometrist will have suitable equipment for this.

Many people who have sustained brain injuries report the loss of a driving licence as the most disabling aspect of their inability to be independent (Pearlman and Fyvie, 1988). Driving after brain damage is a complex topic, and depends in part on the legal requirements of different countries. Vision-related regulations may be based on visual fields, acuity and binocularity, and may differ for private and vocational motorists. This has been discussed in detail by Shute and Woodhouse (1990). Co-operation with other professionals involved in the patient's care is vital, since optometric assessment should form part of a general appraisal of the patient's fitness to drive. Assessment by a clinical psychologist is desirable, since higher-order visual functioning appears to be particularly relevant for road accidents (Charman, 1985), and comprehensive testing on the roads is an essential complement to tests of vision, motor capacity and so on (Jones et al., 1983).

Readers interested in further information about the ways in which cortical lesions can disrupt visual functions, including movement, colour, form, depth amd location, are referred to Wilson et al. (1989).

Conclusions

This chapter has described some of the issues which arise when providing vision care for people with disabilities, including the attitudes which are held in society about such people, as reflected in the kind of language used when referring to them. Background information about a number of conditions was given, including intellectual impairment, hearing impairment, multiple impairments and brain injury. Likely visual problems were outlined, and some appropriate techniques for communicating with patients and assessing their vision described. It was concluded that no patient should be condemned as untestable given the approaches which are possible today.

References

Broadbent H., Westall C. (1989). An evaluation of techniques for measuring stereopsis in infants and young children. *Ophthalmic Physiol. Optics*, 1, 3–7.

Chandna A., Karki C., Davis J., Doran R.M.L. (1989). Preferential looking in the mentally handicapped. *Eye*, **3**, 833–9.

Charman W.N. (1985). Visual standards for driving. *Ophthalmic Physiol. Optics*, **5**, 211–20.

Cockburn D. (1983). Signs and symptoms of stroke and impending stroke in a series of optometric patients. *Am. J. Optom. Physiol. Opt.*, **60**, 749–53.

Comer R.J., Piliavin J.A. (1972). The effects of physical deviance on face-to-face interaction: the other side. *J. Pers. Soc. Psychol.*, **23**, 33–9.

Conrad R. (1981). Sign language in education: some consequent problems. In *Perspectives on BSL and Deafness* (Woll B., Kyle J.G., Deuchar M., eds). London: Croom Helm.

Cress P.J., Spellman C.R., DeBriere T.J. et al. (1981). Vision screening for persons with severe handicaps. *JASH*, **6**, 41.

Dever J. (1988). Hegemony and handicap—a sociological study of disability. Undergraduate thesis, University of Glasgow.

Duckman R.H., Selenow A. (1983). Use of forced preferential looking for measurement of visual acuity in a population of neurologically impaired children. *Am. J. Optom. Physiol. Opt.*, **60**, 817–21.

Freeman C.F., Rudge N.B. (1988). Cerebrovascular accident and the orthoptist. *Br. Orthoptic J.*, **45**, 8–18.

Gianutsos R., Matheson P. (1987). The rehabilitation of visual perceptual disorders attributable to brain injury. In *Neuropsychological Rehabilitation* (Meier M.J., Benton A.L., Diller L., eds). Edinburgh: Churchill Livingstone.

Harries D. (1989). Multi-handicapped people and service development. *Br. J. Visual Impairment*, **VII**, 43–6.

Harrison W. (1985). Assessment and stimulation of vision in multiple-handicapped children. *Br. Orthoptic J.*, **42**, 26–31.

Hertz B.G. (1987). Acuity card testing of retarded children. *Behav. Brain Res.*, **24**, 85–92.

Hertz B.G. (1988). Use of the acuity card method to test retarded children in special schools. *Child: Care, Health Dev.*, **14**, 189–98.

Hertz B.G., Rosenberg J. (1988). Acuity card testing of spastic children: prelminary results. *J. Pediatr. Ophthalmol. Strabismus*, **25**, 139–44.

Hill J.L. (1987). Rights of low vision children and their parents. *Can. J. Optom.*, Summer 1987, **49**, 78–82.

Jacobson L. (1988). Ophthalmology in mentally retarded adults. *Acta Ophthalmol.*, **66**, 457–62.

Jones R., Giddens H., Croft, D. (1983). Assessment and training of brain-damaged drivers. *Am. J. Occup. Ther.*, **37**, 754–60.

Karp A. (1984). Hearing impairment. In *Clinical Low Vision* (Faye E., ed.). Boston: Little, Brown.

Lewis V. (1987). *Development and Handicap*. Oxford: Blackwell.

Lindstedt E. (1986). Early vision assessment in visually impaired children at the TRC, Sweden. *Br. J. Visual Impairment*, **IV**, 49–51.

Lovie-Kitchin J.E., Bowman R.J. (1985). *Senile Macular Degeneration: Management and Rehabilitation*. Boston: Butterworths.

Meades J., Woodhouse J.M., Leat S.J. (1990). Assessment of accommodation in children. *Ophthalmic Physiol. Opt.*, **10**, 413.

Miller E. (1984). *Recovery and Management of Neuropsychological Impairments*. Chichester: Wiley.

Newcombe F. (1985). Rehabilitation in clinical neurology: neuropsychological aspects. In *Handbook of Clinical Neurology* vol.2 (Frederiks J.A.M., ed.). Amsterdam: Elsevier Science, pp. 609–42.

Nooney T.W. (1986). Partial visual rehabilitation of hemianopic patients. *Am. J. Optom. Physiol. Opt.*, **63**, 382–6.

Orel-Bixler D., Haegerstrom-Portnoy G., Hall A. (1989). Visual assessment of the multiply handicapped patient. *Optom. Vision Sci.*, **66**, 530–6.

Pearlman K., Fyvie C. (1988). Running a group for stroke victims: issues and evaluations. Presented at BPS DCP Summer School, July, 1988.

Puzio F.P. (1984). Special ideas for special patients. *Rev. Optom.*, Feb. 1984, 31–2.

Rabbitt R. (1988). Social psychology, neurosciences and cognitive psychology need each other (and gerontology needs all three of them). *Psychologist*, **1**, 500–6.

Rogow S.M., Hass J., Humphries C. (1984). Learning to look: cognitive aspects of visual attention. *Can. J. Optom.*, **46**, 31–4.

Shentall G.A., Hosking G. (1986). A study of the visual defects detected in children with cerebral palsy and children with Down's syndrome. *Br. Orthoptic J.*, **43**, 22–5.

Shute R., Curtis K. (1989). Dysphasia therapy: a respectable occupation? In *Developments in Clinical and Experimental Neuropsychology* (Crawford J.R., Parker D.M., eds). New York: Plenum.

Shute R.H., Woodhouse J.M. (1990). Visual fitness to drive after stroke or head injury. *Ophthalmic Physiol. Optics*, **10**, 327–32.

Smith P.K., Cowie H. (1988). *Understanding Children's Development*. Oxford: Blackwell.

Suchman R.G. (1968). Visual impairment among deaf children. *Volta Rev.*, **70**, 31–7.

Sunderland A., Wade D.T., Hewer R.L. (1987). The natural history of visual neglect after stroke. *Int. Disability Studies*, **9**, 55–9.

Tyerman A. (1989). Self concepts and psychological adjustment after severe head injury. Paper presented to International Conference on Health Psychology, Cardiff, September, 1989.

Verma S. (1988). When the patient is hearing impaired. *Rev. Optom.*, Feb 1988, 78.

Wade D.T., Wood V., Hewer R.L. (1988). Recovery of cognitive function soon after stroke: a study of visual neglect, attention span and verbal recall. *J. Neurol. Neurosurg. Psychiatry*, **51**, 10–13.

Warburg M. (1964). The need for spectacles among mentally retarded persons. In *International Copenhagen Congress for the Scientific Study of Mental Retardation* vol. 2 (Oster J., ed.). pp. 779–82.

Warburg M. (1970). Tracing and training of blind and partially sighted patients in institutions for the mentally retarded. *Dan. Med. Bull.*, **17**, 148–52.

Warburg M. (1982). Why are blind and severely visually impaired children with mental retardation much more retarded than sighted children? Symposium on early visual development. *Acta Ophthalmol. (Copenh)*, **157**, (suppl.) 72–81.

Weinmann J. (1987). *An Outline of Psychology as Applied to Medicine*. Bristol: Wright.

Wilson B. (1989). Models of cognitive rehabilitation. In *Models of Brain-injury Rehabilitation* (Eames P., Wood R., eds). London: Croom Helm.

Wilson J.T.L., Dutton G.N., Wiedmann K.D. (1989). Neuropsychological evidence for localisation of visual sensory functions. In *Developments in Clinical and Experimental Neuropsychology* (Crawford J.R., Parker D.M., eds). New York: Plenum.

Woodruff M.E. (1977). Prevalence of visual and ocular anomalies in 168 non-institutionalized mentally retarded children. *Can. J. Public Health*, **68**, 225–32.

Woodruff M.E. (1986). Differential effects of various causes of deafness on the eyes, refractive errors, and vision of children. *Am. J. Ophthalmol. Physiol. Opt.*, **63**, 668–75.

Chapter 8

Psychological aspects of visual impairment

Introduction

Terminology

The usage of terms such as 'blind' and 'partially sighted' can be a source of confusion amongst both professional and lay people who come into contact with those who have severely impaired vision. Definitions have been drawn up for medical and legal purposes; for example, in the USA legal blindness is maximum acuity 20/200 and/or maximum field 20°. However, such categorization may not be reflected in the ways individuals actually function in visual terms: two people with similar ocular conditions and similar low visual acuity may operate quite differently from one another. Barraga (1976) pointed out that visual functioning is related only in part to the condition of the eye, and is 'determined by the experiences, motivations, needs and expectations of each individual in relation to whatever visual capacity is available to satisfy curiosity and accomplish activities for personal satisfaction'. This emphasizes the central importance of psychological factors in understanding visual impairment.

With reference to education, Chapman and Stone (1988) have proposed that the word 'blind' should be reserved for those with no vision at all or with light perception only, since labelling people as 'blind' will discourage them, and those working with them, from making the most of their remaining visual capacity. A case in point was described in the previous chapter, where a girl labelled as blind had not been undertaking any visually-based learning at school, although she turned out to have a corrected monocular acuity of 6/45. Another example is the case of a boy attending a school for blind children who, when asked to read a piece of text, said, 'I'm blind—I can't do this', yet, when encouraged to try, he read N24 print size at 20 cm, unaided (Leat, personal communication). Labelling those with residual vision as blind also means that they may be inappropriately directed to services for the totally blind; Genensky (1976) has emphasized the importance of distinguishing between legal and functional blindness in this respect.

Chapman and Stone (1988) have also discussed the phrases 'visually limited' and 'partially sighted'. 'Visually limited' is a term often used in the USA to refer to pupils who use their vision for all school tasks, albeit with prescribed lenses and special lighting conditions. 'Partially sighted', besides being a legal category, is often used to refer to pupils who use vision for all tasks, but where special educational materials and adaptations are required. A reservation they have about the use of this term is that it is frequently used in contrast with 'blind', a dichotomy which ignores the needs of children who utilize both tactile and visual methods for learning.

The term 'low vision' is a general one useful in both clinical practice and education to include those with visual difficulties, whether or not registered as legally blind or partially sighted, who may benefit from specialized visual assessment, advice, low vision aids or educational interventions.

Terminology has also been discussed by Lovie-Kitchin and Bowman (1985), in connection with senile macular degeneration (age-related maculopathy) and their discussion has a wider relevance to the field of disability, as mentioned in the introduction to the previous chapter. They drew a distinction between visual impairment, disability and handicap. Impairment is a limitation of one or more of the basic visual functions: if visual aids provide compensation, a disability is then said not to exist. Disability occurs when an impairment results in a limitation of ability to perform certain tasks: it depends on degree of impairment and the tasks the person has to perform, such as reading, writing, orientation and mobility. Handicap is the disadvantage a person experiences because of a disability: it depends on the disability, the person's expectations and those of others, and the demands of the environment; it may include loss of independence, self-esteem, friends and job.

The role of the optometrist in low vision

Hill (1987) has suggested that eye professionals too often have the attitude that they are interested in vision but have little interest in blindness. However, the optometrist has a central role to play at the stages of impairment and disability, initially in the detection of ocular anomalies and referral for ophthalmological investigation and possible treatment, and then in reducing the visual disability by normal optometric prescriptions, low vision aids and the giving of advice about lighting conditions, other special services and so on.

Lovie-Kitchin and Bowman (1985) see the reduction of handicap as being the province of other professionals, such as social workers and psychologists, and advocate referral to such other rehabilitation professionals when appropriate. As will be discussed further later, however, the optometrist also has a part to play in reducing handicap, by encouraging high self-esteem in patients and fostering their ability to cope with their reduced vision.

There is an increasing demand for low vision services, as demographic changes mean that age-related visual loss is becoming more common. Those over the age of 65 are over-represented in the population with severe visual dysfunction, in comparison with their numbers in the general population. For example, in this age group, cataracts and glaucoma are eight times more common than in the general population while, in functional terms, 5% have visual impairments severe enough to prevent the reading of ordinary newsprint, even with refractive corrections.

These older patients are much more likely to be female, which probably reflects the greater life expectancy of women. However, examining the elderly population as a whole, a preponderance of men report visual loss as the main cause of their limitation in activity, and at one particular low vision clinic more men than women attended (Leat and Rumney, 1990). These findings are thought to reflect not a difference in visual functioning per se between the sexes, but a greater likelihood that men will perceive the same level of visual loss as handicapping (Birren and Williams, 1982). This may reflect differential social demands placed on men, it may mean that women cope better with low vision, or that they have lower expectations (they may put up with health problems without complaint). There is, in fact, some evidence that women adjust to disability better than men (Carson, 1990).

There are, then, increasing numbers of elderly patients with low vision, and it has been estimated that there are many who could benefit from specialized optometric care but are not being referred for it (Kirchner and Philips, 1980). In addition, the incidence of severe visual impairment in infants is thought to be increasing, partly because more very premature babies and children with perinatal complications are being saved. Low vision therefore seems to be a field of optometry set for expansion, and some optometrists may seek to specialize in it. An understanding of the role of vision in a person's developmental tasks is very important, as *functional* vision lies at the heart of low vision practice. In young patients, the role their residual vision can play in their social, motor and cognitive development must be understood, particularly so that the optometrist will have insight into the kinds of rehabilitation processes and their aims that others working with the child, such as teachers, special needs advisers and physiotherapists, may have. While children with low vision may only occasionally come to the attention of those who do not specialize, all optometrists will regularly meet older patients with failing vision, and need to understand the psychological implications this has, and the part that good vision care can play in helping people to retain their independence.

The adjustment to being partially sighted, for both the youngster and the older person, may be even more difficult than to being totally blind, as these individuals are in a kind of limbo between the blind and sighted worlds, often desperately trying to appear normal (Tuttle, 1984). People with poor vision in both eyes (not correctable to better than 20/50) tend to have reduced feelings of self-worth, diminished emotional security and restricted leisure, group and work activities (Anderson and Palmore, 1974). Furthermore, Snyder et al. (1976) found indications of poor mental status in association with poor vision, although it was unclear whether poor vision caused low mental status or whether both were associated with other factors, such as degenerative disease. Older low vision patients are likely to have additional physical problems, and severe visual impairment is more common in low-income families (Kirchner and Peterson, 1979). It does seem, therefore, that the low vision population is one where a high proportion of patients will have a range of social and psychological problems to which the vision care specialist needs to be sensitive.

Stereotypes and visual impairment

In an earlier chapter, there was discussion of the phenomenon of stereotyping, which leads to people interacting with a stereotyped individual in ways which are inappropriate and insulting. People with visual handicaps appear to be subject to such processes, although there is relatively little research on this (Coupland et al., 1986). What evidence there is suggests that 'the blind' are seen as non-accepted and isolated, as helpless and dependent, and as needing help from the sighted, and visually impaired people often report that such social stigmas are worse than the loss of vision itself. As will be discussed further later, the sighted often assume that those with severe visual impairments are more depressed than is actually the case. Such stereotypes are based in part on ignorance of the true diversity that exists among the visually impaired. The sighted fail to distinguish between those with congenital as opposed to acquired impairments, or those whose vision is lost gradually through degenerative conditions rather than suddenly, as in the case of accident. They may assume that someone who is registered as blind can see nothing at all, whereas they may have some residual vision. In addition, the sighted may experience that general discomfort which the able-bodied feel in interacting with those with disabilities, and see the individual as blind first and a person second (see introduction to the previous chapter).

The types of language which people use to one another reflect the roles that they perceive themselves and others to have, and it seems that those with visual impairments tend to receive linguistic messages from the sighted which cast them into the stereotypical roles just described. It is commonplace, for example, for people to talk about them in their presence, as though they were not present ('Does he take sugar?'), or to use language styles which amount to talking down to them. It has been suggested that repeatedly being on the receiving end of such types of communication can induce feelings of helplessness and low self-worth, so that people with visual impairments eventually come to see themselves as handicapped (a similar process was noted in Chapter 5 with reference to the way younger people talk down to the elderly). Blindness has been referred to as a 'learned social role', and may in turn perpetuate the existing stereotypes—a cyclical social process. The way a person reacts to visual loss which occurs suddenly may be influenced by such stereotypes: they may live up (or down) to their own stereotypical image of the blind (Dodds, 1988). Later in this chapter we will examine ways in which the optometrist can help to break the mould of helplessness in their visually impaired patients.

Early visual impairment

As noted earlier, it is widely believed that the numbers of children being born with visual impairments in western society is growing (Ferrell, 1984). There are a number of probable reasons for this. Firstly, there are more girls who are becoming mothers in their early teens, when there is a greater risk of complications such as low birth weight, which greatly increases the chance of visual and other problems in the baby. At the other end of the spectrum, more women are putting off having babies until late in their reproductive years, again increasing the risk of birth defects. In addition, premature babies are being saved at earlier and earlier stages of gestation, again with an associated higher risk of visual impairments; in fact, a second epidemic of retinopathy of prematurity has been reported (Kolata, 1986).

Prematurity

Premature babies, those born before 37 weeks or weighing less than 2500 g or 5½ lb), often have particular problems and developmental patterns that differ from those of full-term infants. With modern care, babies born as much as 3 months early, weighing less than 1 kg, can survive, but the incidence of permanent problems is greater the less mature the infant was at birth. Neurological problems may arise, which seem to result from general circulatory problems: there is rupture of the fragile capillaries around the brain ventricles, resulting in intraventricular haemorrhage. If this is mild, there is no permanent damage, and the infant may eventually be indistinguishable from a full-term baby, but if it is severe the infant may die, or survive with cerebral palsy and intellectual impairment.

Not much is known about the relationship between neurological problems and visual development, but it seems that if there is ventricular dilation and periventricular haemorrhage, severe visual deficits are likely. When it first became possible to save the lives of premature babies in the 1950s and 1960s, there was a high incidence of retinopathy of prematurity, due at least in part to oxygen levels which were too high, leading to neovascularization of the retina, particularly in the periphery, sometimes resulting in retrolental fibroplasia. The incidence dropped as oxygen levels became subject to more careful monitoring, but there seems to be an increase again in recent years. It is not entirely clear why this is so, but it may be partly because younger and younger babies are surviving with improved care. Myopia, astigmatism and strabismus are other possible consequences of prematurity.

Premature children are likely to remain small until 5 or 6 years of age. In general, they tend to obtain lower scores on cognitive and motor developmental tests during the first 5 years, and those from economically deprived backgrounds have the lowest scores of all. Some are more restless and distractable than normal, and there is a higher incidence of hyperactivity, autism and accident-proneness, and also of later child abuse.

Most catch up by about 4 years, however, and there are generally significant impairments in IQ only in some very low birthweight babies who have had additional problems. Some problems do seem to be due to prematurity per se, but there may be other reasons, such as birth complications, multiple births and the abnormal early environment: being in an incubator is neither like being in the uterus nor like a normal postnatal environment. As a result of the abnormal social circumstances, and sometimes feelings of guilt and disappointment in the parents, parental behaviour and attitudes may be affected: the mother may hold the baby at a distance instead of cuddling it, and some feel less attached to their baby even months later. Stimulation of premature infants, for example, playing heart beat recordings and rocking them, has resulted in more advanced sensory and motor skills and exploratory behaviour, at least in the short term. The later environment is also important for alleviating any early damage and, if there are visual deficits, the optometrist can play a part in this.

Visual impairment and early development

Other major causes of severe visual difficulties in infants in the developed world are optic atrophy and cataracts, frequently as a result of maternal rubella in pregnancy. Approaches to severe congenital visual impairment, whatever its origin, have changed in recent years. While at one time it was usual to send children away to residential schools for the blind when school entry age was reached, with minimal involvement of parents, now many more are educated in mainstream schools, and the important role of parents as rehabilitators, especially in the early preschool years, is now acknowledged (Leung and Hollins, 1989).

Hill (1987) has made essentially the same point as Chapman and Stone (1988), that a distinction must be made between the blind and the partially-sighted child: children with even minimal vision are nevertheless children with vision and, in line with the idea that blindness is an acquired social role, there is a danger that they may taught to be 'blind' not just by the attitudes of the general public but by the types of services that are provided. It is especially important for parents to be told about the level of residual vision if the child is registerable as blind.

Hill maintains that the most basic right of the low vision child is that of accurate diagnosis of the problem, yet there is evidence that children are often diagnosed as cortically blind without confirmatory electrophysiological evidence (Allen and Fraser, 1983). Children may also fail to receive appropriate rehabilitative interventions. For example, Hofstetter (1985) examined the needs of 60 students in Indiana diagnosed as having a significant visual loss: 45% would certainly have benefited from special visual aids and rehabilitative guidance, and a high additional percentage would probably have done so; in addition, almost a half with refractive corrections did not have appropriate prescriptions. Similarly, Leat and Karadsheh (1991) have reported that many visually impaired children, both in mainstream special units and in schools for the blind in England and Wales, are not being supplied with appropriate low vision aids, nor given sufficient help to cope with the aids they have. Hill notes: 'Eye practitioners must act as advocates for this unique population.' Referring to the Canadian situation, she says that there is an urgent need for low vision practitioners to serve the needs of these children.

That vision plays a central role in normal development was emphasized in Chapter 5, where it was pointed out that children with severe visual impairments are often delayed in many areas. It is important to note at this point, however, that many of the studies on this were carried out when less was known about normal developmental processes, in the days before parents were encouraged to become actively involved in promoting their children's development, and it is anticipated that there will soon have to be a revision of developmental norms for blind children (Leung and Hollins, 1989). It must not bè assumed, therefore, that children with visual impairments will inevitably lag behind their peers in development. Nor must average attainment necessarily be considered adequate, as children with high IQs have the potential to perform at levels above the average. The optometrist can play a role in helping children to fulfil their potential by assessing their visual strengths and weaknesses and providing advice and visual aids aimed at making the most of any residual vision.

When interacting with an infant with severe visual impairment, it can be unnerving if the child displays no eye contact and reduced facial expressiveness. However, Fraiberg (1977) noted that the usual facial signals between adult and baby can be replaced by equivalent touch signals (fingering the face and then stopping fingering being equivalent to gazing and looking away). Parents' attention can be drawn to such patterns to help facilitate social and language development, helping the child to develop the concept of 'turn-taking' in conversation, something often absent in 'conversations' between blind babies and their parents, as the parent often monopolizes the interaction. The optometrist should be aware of this: in situations where he or she would be chatting with a fully sighted infant or toddler to establish rapport, the youngster with a visual impairment should be allowed to touch.

Babies with severe visual impairments show a fear of strangers at the same age as other infants, and the optometrist should be prepared for exactly the same problems as with a sighted baby around 7 months or older: the child may initially be very wary of a stranger's voice, and object strongly to being held by someone new, but will probably be happy to interact with them if on the lap of a parent or other carer. However, in another related respect, blind babies may have to be handled differently. A sighted toddler displays a normal separation anxiety when a parent leaves, and one would not normally be expecting to test a small child's vision without the parent being present. Blind babies, however, display this separation anxiety at a later age; they seem to be delayed in coming to realize that objects which disappear still exist and can reappear. The upshot is that a 12-month-old blind baby may be undisturbed if the parent leaves the room; however, once separation anxiety does develop, it may go on until a later age than usual, and the child may become exceptionally distressed if he or she realizes that the parent is not present. It is important, therefore, to be prepared for a small child with severe visual impairment to be 'clingier' than usual, and the optometrist should not make prejudicial judgements such as assuming that the parents have been overprotective.

As discussed in Chapter 5, visually impaired children may lag behind in their motor development and exploratory behaviour, if vision is not sufficient to motivate these behaviours. Rehabilitation involves making the visual modality attractive, with large, brightly coloured and shiny toys, and encouraging the child's motor behaviour. For example, sitting can be encouraged by propping the baby up with pillows or a special baby chair, a room can be made safe for exploration by using safety gates and padding sharp furniture, and the child can be encouraged to walk by standing on the parent's feet while the parent walks backwards; the use of the hands is encouraged by giving the child toys to manipulate and playing clapping games. By providing a full assessment of the child's visual capabilities, the optometrist can cooperate with those working with the child, saying, for example, whether central vision is normal, whether there are field losses, and the implications these factors are likely to have for what the child can reasonably be expected to do, such as the degree of detail the child will be able to see and the likely effects on mobility.

The importance of interprofessional co-operation is recognized at the Tomteboda Resource Centre for Visually Handicapped Children in Sweden, described by Lindstedt (1986). A team care approach is used, the optometrist working alongside an ophthalmologist, psychologist, special teacher and human factors engineer. The child's visual assessment is thus an integrated part of the total developmental assessment of the child, and helps in the formation of a rehabilitation programme. Courses for parents are also offered at the centre. The centre tends to concentrate increasingly on the youngest children, in view of the present state of knowledge about early visual development and the role of vision for early general development.

Education

As children reach school age, educational concerns come to the fore, and optometric input is useful in decision-making about whether braille, vision or a mixture of methods should be used, and in the provision of aids to maximize the visual capability that the child has. Interprofessional co-operation is again important, as stressed by Hill (1987). If a child is provided with a low vision aid, but the teachers are not told about its use and there is no follow-up, it is likely to remain unused in a drawer.

Education about the condition itself and the available services should be provided, and this is one facet of the role of the optometrist, as discussed in an earlier chapter. The parents of a child with visual impairment often know very little about the condition. For example, they may be able to say that the child has had an operation, but be unable to say precisely what the nature of it was. Also, they may not realize if the condition is a genetic one, and Hill points out that they, and later the children themselves, are entitled to genetic counselling, as well as vocational guidance to avoid the building up of plans which are unrealistically high or low.

Teenagers may become self-conscious about the appearance of visual aids such magnifiers and telescopes and reject them, so alternatives such as closed circuit television and the use of taped notes may have to be used until the young person feels ready to use other methods again. The low vision adviser must be aware of the cosmetic implications of aids and discuss them with young patients; if this aspect is ignored, the end-result will be non-compliance by the patient (Faye et al., 1984). A young person who refuses to use a low vision aid at school can still be encouraged to use it at home.

The importance of listening to the point of view of the patient has been stressed throughout this book. This is particularly important with patients with disabilities in order to avoid a patronizing attitude (related to being *in* authority rather than *an* authority—see Chapter 3). Unfortunately, people with disabilities have rarely been asked for their own views. An exception to this is the work of Tobin and Hill (1987, 1988, 1989) about the concerns of teenagers with visual impairments. This was part of a longitudinal study of 120 blind and partially sighted children attending special schools in England and Wales, most being diagnosed as visually impaired before they were 1 year old. Sixty-eight per cent favoured education in special schools, because of small classes, individual attention, special facilities and equipment, and specially qualified teachers, although the disadvantages were isolation from the sighted world and few friends in their home districts. Thirty-one per cent intended to go into the helping professions, and a fifth planned commercial or industrial careers. Fifty-two per cent definitely planned to marry and have a family, while 5% intended not to do so. Fifty-five per cent enjoyed listening to music, while other popular activities included swimming, rock-climbing and canoeing.

The majority of the teenagers accepted their visual situation well and with humour, and did not see a cure for blindness as being as important as a cure for cancer. The attitudes of fully sighted people which they reported ranged from being very helpful (although sometimes patronizing) to horrendously cruel, as when sighted youngsters told them it was safe to cross the road when vehicles were coming. Over half reported being called names or regarded as mentally retarded by other children. The teenagers were keen for attitudinal change and education among the general public, through schools and the media. Taking a wider perspective, many of the group reported anxiety about possible nuclear war, and in this they are typical of other teenagers.

This study demonstrates that youngsters with visual impairments are generally well adjusted and in most respects like their sighted peers, with various interests, ambitions and concerns, and with a dislike of being patronized. All this underlines the message that the optometrist should find out the particular concerns and activities of all their patients; as the British youngsters just described demonstrate, it would be quite wrong to assume that those with severe visual impairments spend their time quietly in armchairs!

Later visual loss

Reactions to visual loss

In keeping with the lifespan perspective outlined in Chapter 5, Robbins and McMurray (1988) have described loss of vision as a non-normative life event. Although most people will experience some reduction in the efficiency of their visual functioning as they grow older, the majority do not experience severe loss of vision, whether gradual or sudden. Such a non-normative event will be responded to differently by different people, and may itself be the trigger for personality change. Robbins and McMurray found a correlation between poor vision and a personality variable known as hardiness (discussed further below). One interpretation is that visual loss triggers change, but since causality cannot be assumed from a correlation, there is also the possibility that certain personality types are more prone to the condition under consideration (age-related maculopathy) than others, perhaps mediated by stress-related physiological changes.

Shindell (1988) has discussed reactions to diabetic retinopathy, something which is likely to cause a gradual loss of vision, but which may have been anticipated for a long time. It may also have a more wide-ranging significance in indicating that the general health of the patient is deteriorating. A particular problem which Shindell identifies is that low vision does not lend itself to easy understanding by other people: it is invisible, varies between patients, and is difficult for family and friends to understand. This lack of understanding extends to professionals also; depression is over-reported when either family or professionals describe people with disabilities. This seems to stem from the fact that others try to imagine how they would feel under the circumstances, but only

think as far ahead as the immediate impact of visual loss, forgetting that adjustment does occur. In reality, the incidence of
depression found in rehabilitation centres is only 5–
15%.

Many visually impaired people who divorce blame the divorce on
the disability, but studies show that the divorce rate is no higher
than in the rest of the population (Shindell, 1988). Problems such
as visual loss can weaken a weak relationship, but can also
strengthen a basically sound one. Rates of suicide and alcohol abuse
are also comparable with figures for the general population. Often,
psychological difficulty is manifested not at the sight loss itself, but
at the accompanying social confusion. Losing one's vision affects a
person's self-concept, which must go through a process of change
and result in a new self-concept which incorporates acceptance of
the visual loss; however, since the partially sighted often have
particular difficulty because of the limbo situation in which they find
themselves, many with diabetic retinopathy find themselves with an
ambiguous self-image, neither blind nor sighted. They may also find
themselves isolated as family and friends disengage or distance
themselves, perhaps out of fear that the person will die, or that they
will upset them by saying the wrong things.

An individual's response to his or her loss of vision is often
described as a bereavement-type of process, in which the person
passes through a series of stages. This is something which has been
described as happening in response to a range of life crises, such as
the death of a loved one (the original context in which it was
studied) or the diagnosis of a life-threatening disease (Kubler-Ross,
1969). The first stage is shock, during which the situation may be
denied or minimized. Then there may be a period of reactive
depression (a natural response to traumatic happenings), followed
by readjustment as the person accepts the situation and learns to
cope with it. There may not be a smooth progression from one stage
to the next, in fact, but the person may swing back and forth. It is
generally maintained that those who show a strong initial grief
reaction and are able to express their feelings are able to make the
best psychological adjustment in the long term.

This bereavement model has been very influential in considering
life crises, but it has been criticized by Dodds (1989), on a number
of grounds. Firstly, workers in low vision claim that the sequence
of emotional responses described does not occur in reality, despite
the superficial plausibility. Secondly, the process is untestable, since
if someone does not express a predicted emotion they are said to
have repressed it, and it will need to be worked through at a later
date (there is a psychoanalytic influence here). Thirdly, the loss
model implies that intervention cannot take place until the person
has worked through certain emotions and is ready for it.

Dodds (1989) puts forward an alternative model for understanding sudden visual loss, based on self-efficacy, a notion which was mentioned in Chapter 4 in connection with the health belief model. Dodds proposes that the person is plunged into a state of incompetence, which leads to a loss of self-esteem and depression, which will prevent him or her from participating in rehabilitative activity. This model has different implications from the loss model, in that it suggests that the person should become involved in rehabilitative activity at an early stage in order to regain competence, rather than withdrawing from activity to work through certain emotions.

This proposal ties in with a suggestion made by Robbins and McMurray. In their study of people with age-related maculopathy, activities of daily living were measured, giving a score indicating the degree to which the person is able to carry out ordinary aspects of everyday life, such as dressing, reading and mobility. It was found that the person was more depressed if there was a lower score. Again, cause and effect cannot be assumed—either the person was unable to perform activities because of depression, or they were depressed because of becoming incapable. The authors assume that the latter is a possibility, and propose that if the low vision specialist can improve the person's functioning, as reflected in the activities of daily living score, then depression is likely to lift also.

Dodds takes Bandura's self-efficacy theory as the basis of this alternative, competence-based model (Bandura, 1977). It concerns the way an individual views his or her own competence, these perceptions being derived from a number of sources. Firstly, there is the appraisal of one's own performance, of past successes and failures. Secondly, there is information gained from the performance of others in a similar situation to oneself—in this context, other visually impaired people. Thirdly, the stress of trying to perform a difficult task can lead to future avoidance, and a further reduction of self-efficacy. Finally, there is the question of how the rehabilitator attributes success or failure: if success is attributed to the ability of the patient, and failure to factors outside his or her control, such as task difficulty, rather than to, say, lack of effort, then self-efficacy will be raised. This is related to the notion of locus of control (discussed further below), whereby events are seen to be within or outside one's own control. Self-efficacy is also seen as a route to maintaining high self-esteem.

This model has yet to be tested in the context of low vision, but Dodds offers it as a possible alternative to the loss model. These considerations for the rehabilitator are not just confined to the case of visual loss: similar factors are relevant when dealing with a whole range of patients who must come to terms with difficult circumstances, whether it is recovering from a stroke or coping with a baby with multiple impairments.

People whose visual loss is the result of cataracts may have particular worries as they await surgery. Little consideration has been given to this, despite the fact that it is the most common surgical procedure performed on people aged 65 or older. The emotional aspects of cataract surgery were examined by O'Malley et al. (1989) in a retro-spective study which looked at understanding of the procedure and anxiety surrounding it in 14 patients (mean age 85 years). Although several patients reported some brightening of mood after the operation as a result of being able to appreciate colours and so on, no actual mourning for sight, as predicted by the loss model, was reported while they were awaiting surgery; this may have been because they regarded the loss as temporary. The vast majority could not give basic information about what the procedure had entailed, and were unable to point out the lens on a model eye. Fourteen per cent wanted technical information about the operation, while 36% did not; 28% found technical information anxiety-provoking. This creates prob-lems for the idea that informed consent for surgery should be obtained, as it actually increased anxiety in some patients. As has been found in studies of children's responses to medical procedures, it is not the most obvious aspects of surgery, such as cutting the eye, which were most anxiety-provoking, but staying immobile, hearing surgeons talking during the procedure, and concerns about whether the operation would be a success; in addition, a few patients were worried by surgical drapes, fear of breaking the incision, concerns over other medical problems, fear of the intraocular procedure itself and having an acquaintance with poor results from similar surgery. Ways of dealing with these worries will be discussed later.

Locus of control

That a feeling of being able to control events oneself (having an internal locus of control) is important in low vision rehabilitation has been shown by Robbins and McMurray (1988), in their study of psychological and visual factors in age-related maculopathy. They recognized that the nature of the visual loss does not in itself predict how well the patient will do, since the person's perception of the event may be more important. They drew on the more general psychological literature on stress and coping, which suggests that those who cope well with stress are *hardy* (Kobasa, 1979), characterized by a sense of control over life events, an involved commitment to self and others and a sense that change presents a challenge rather than a threat. Such a person, it is also argued, will make good use of social resources, such as friends and money, at their disposal (Kobasa and Pucetti, 1983).

Robbins and McMurray postulated that low vision patients with a hardy personality would be more likely to benefit from rehabilitation.

They found that success at rehabilitation was best predicted by personality hardiness, age and low-contrast acuity—the younger (of this elderly group), hardier patients with better residual vision were better able to use rehabilitation resources to cope with the adjustment to low vision.

They also found evidence which suggested that an internal locus of control with regard to health might be relinquished as a result of experience of age-related maculopathy, and likened this to a similar finding in long-term diabetics. It seems that some people who once saw their health as being under their own control lose this perception when a devastating change in health status comes along. Their findings also suggested that there may be a reduction of belief in the ability of powerful others to control health. It seems likely that these changes arise as the patient becomes aware that neither they nor their medical advisers have any control over the disease process.

The question of enabling patients to take, or regain, control has been discussed in some depth by Gardner and McCormack (1990). They quote a number of health-related areas where research has indicated that when people start to believe in their own capability, and are given the freedom to exercise these beliefs in action, then health improvements occur; the areas where this has been demonstrated include stress control, dealing with low back pain and introducing dietary changes in adolescence. However, passing control over to patients should not be done too quickly, they say: good communication skills are needed to gauge the views of the patient in this respect and take account of them.

The same point has been made by Dodds with specific reference to low vision. He points out that some of these people will have become 'patientized' in the passive sense discussed in Chapter 3, and may expect decisions to be made for them. This is likely to be especially true of elderly people, who may have low expectations of what they can do, and see a visual impairment as the last straw in a sequence of events indicating deteriorating health. The low vision adviser, he says, may be the first person to act in an enabling role although, paradoxically, he or she may have to act as advocate for the patient initially against his or her own preconceptions or prejudices. All the lessons about communication and taking the patient's point of view into account (Chapter 4) apply with particular force when it comes to dealing with patients who have low vision.

Encouraging self-efficacy

Dodds's model of visual loss, based on Bandura's self-efficacy theory, has implications for rehabilitation. It suggests that intervention should be early, rather than late, to avoid the person falling into a state of learned helplessness (Seligman, 1975). The patient needs to be able to monitor success, and this involves setting goals which are clear, reachable and not too far in the distance. The involvement of well functioning visually impaired people with whom the individual can identify may provide useful models, also.

Encouraging patients to monitor and believe in their own abilities must start right from the original visual assessment. Padula (1982) has described how the examiner can stimulate motivation, interest and co-operation by designing the examination so that the patient can perform successfully. For example, a standard Snellen chart should not be used as it will reinforce the idea of failure. Instead, a special low vision chart should be available, which has larger letters and can be used at any distance at which the person can see. There should be good lighting to maximize the patient's visual functioning in the test situation. All the normal procedures for examining fields, refractive status and eye health should be adapted to emphasize the particular abilities and positive attributes which the patient retains (this is a particular example of using suitable procedures to avoid anxiety and so forth, as outlined in Chapter 2).

The study by Robbins and McMurray (1988) implies that older patients with poorer residual vision may have greater difficulty in benefiting from rehabilitation, and practitioners need to be aware of the effect of the visual changes on the patient's perceptions, particularly their perceptions of control over their health and eye condition. Care should be taken, therefore, when saying that nothing can be done—while this may be true in the case of the condition itself, things should be phrased more positively, in terms of the prognosis and available rehabilitation resources. Lovie-Kitchin and Bowman (1985) note that most people with age-related maculopathy derive psychological assistance from knowing that they will retain peripheral vision, and hence mobility.

There is, perhaps, a certain conflict between Dodds' suggestion that rehabilitation should begin early to allow the patient to develop strategies for coping with everyday life and the feeling of other writers, particularly those influenced by the loss model, who argue that the patient should be allowed to set his or her own rate of adaptation. This latter strategy perhaps leaves open the possibility that a depressed patient will indeed learn to become helpless. Shindell (1988) warns against using the loss model in a rigid way, pointing out that stresses and changing circumstances can cause people to react as if in an earlier stage, such as becoming depressed; he makes the valid point that such occurrences should not be labelled as 'regressions', since people with visual loss should be entitled to the same range of emotional expression as the able-bodied population. Perhaps the answer is that the professional should be ready to offer practical help and advice right from the start, but should also be ready to deal with negative emotions as they arise at any stage during rehabilitation. It is a question of being able to use the various types of counselling skills, described elsewhere in this book, at the right time. There may be times when a patient does need a little push, perhaps, but this must always be accompanied by setting an attainable goal so that the effort is rewarded and a sense of self-efficacy built up.

It may be difficult for low vision patients to retain a feeling of self-efficacy in the outside world in the face of stereotypical reactions from other people about their needs. A patient who finds this a problem may benefit from referral to a psychologist who will help with social skills training, offering strategies for both asking for and refusing help from other people in an acceptable way. As in the case of people with all kinds of disabilities, those with visual impairments often have to take charge themselves of dealing with the anxiety or misconceptions of other people. Successful rehabilitation involves integrating their disability into how they perceive themselves, accepting the permanent nature of it and focusing on abilities which are open to them rather than on impossible tasks. A patient who has achieved success in rehabilitation may eventually be able to assist others.

Strategies for rehabilitation

One problem, when faced with a patient whose whole life has been turned upside-down by visual loss, is where to begin. Lovie-Kitchin and Bowman (1985) have spelled out priorities in helping a patient to cope with age-related maculopathy. They divide patient needs into two groups—primary and secondary needs. The primary needs are: communication (written and spoken); mobility; home and personal management; emotional and psychological needs. Secondary needs are: recreation; socialization; accommodation; financial; vocational; education; health care; community integration. It might reasonably be argued that these secondary needs are also very important, and in some cases may need to be dealt with urgently. However, the writers' intention in defining primary needs is that they are what is necessary for 'just getting through the day'. They again adopt the premise, which Dodds would support, that simply enabling someone to get through the day will reduce psychological and emotional problems, and set the stage for dealing with other aspects later. The key to successful management, they say, is careful history-taking in order to understand a patient's particular needs, achieved by such methods as asking open-ended questions (if the reader has read this book through from the beginning, this will sound very familiar by now). It is often the practice of low vision clinics to use a questionnaire to gain detailed information about a person's lifestyle and visual needs (Rumney, personal communication).

Cataract patients are rather different from those with untreatable degenerative conditions, since they can look forward to improved vision eventually. First, though, they have to undergo an operation which, as the study described earlier showed, can cause anxiety (O'Malley et al. 1989). The patients in that study had not had their preoperative anxiety assessed, and there had been little attempt to allay it. Factors which tended to alleviate anxiety varied between patients, and included confidence in their ophthalmologist; friends and acquaintances with successful surgery; the availability of immediate postoperative help; experience of previous surgery, including previous cataract surgery; the use of general anaesthetic in some cases; inpatient surgery in some cases and outpatient surgery in others; a second opinion. Suggested remedies are explaining the operative process, not just in terms of the actual operation, which causes more anxiety in some patients, but including the process of being wheeled in and the use of surgical drapes; giving specific details about surgery to those who want it; for surgeons, taking care about what they say during a procedure with a patient who is awake; finally, putting the patient in touch with someone who has had successful cataract surgery may be helpful.

Shindell (1988) has summarized the role of the optometrist in low vision in a way that takes account of many of the psychological points discussed both in this chapter and elsewhere in this book. It can act as a reminder of some of the major points to bear in mind when dealing with patients, of whom people with low vision form a special group.

1. The optometrist acts as an expert consultant. This is related to being *an* authority rather than *in* authority, and to moving the locus of control from practitioner to patient. A paternalistic attitude, whereby the optometrist is personally responsible for the patient's successes and failures, should be avoided. Rather, the optometrist should provide expert care and debunk any myths patients may have about their condition or low vision aids.

2. The optometrist can act as a gatekeeper, keeping informed of local and national resources for patients.

3. The optometrist is in a position to reinforce positive behaviour by the patient.

4. The optometrist should not impose his or her own values, but look at the patient's goals and how they might be attained. The coping style of the professional, such as depending on science or on religion, may not be that of the patient. (The

optometrist may also be able to help a patient to set or clarify goals—Leat, personal comunication.)

5. Shindell advises against seeing denial as automatically bad and to be confronted. It represents the patient's way of dealing with frightening facts. Harshly confronting him or her with the truth may make the practitioner feel good (as though something positive is being done) but will not help the patient. Denial should instead be decreased by presenting the facts, but in a non-frightening manner. Professionals sometimes think that change must be instantaneous, that something need only be said once, that the timing of interventions is irrelevant—all of which are untrue. Sometimes patients go on believing that their sight will miraculously be restored. Shindell says the practitioner should then ask himself or herself, 'Can this person still benefit from my services despite our disagreement about this belief?'

6. Attention should be paid to the process as well as the content of the interaction. A patient may not simply have come for vision care, but for social contact or to please family members. Again, the professional needs to find out why the person has come at this point in time, and what he or she expects to gain.

7. Each patient is unique. The practitioner should resist labelling patients as 'diabetics' or 'cataracts', as if they are wholly defined by their conditions. Each person is an individual dealing with a disease process which is probably frightening for him or her.

The final point is that the professional should ensure understanding between patient and practitioner. The clinician's goal is not simply to act as a technician prescribing visual aids. In keeping with the biopsychosocial approach to health and illness outlined in the opening chapter, the aim of optometric care, as oulined by Shindell (1988) for the case of low vision, and paraphrased here is:

> to aid in improving each patient's quality of life socially, emotionally and behaviourally so that persons see fewer limitations and realistically appraise the options available to them.

Conclusions

This final chapter has outlined some psychological implications of severely impaired vision and the role of the optometrist in reducing resultant disability and handicap. There is a great need for low vision services and, since many patients can be helped with simple aids and low magnification (Leat and Rumney, 1990), they can be assisted within the context of normal optometric practice.

Here, at the end of the book, the reader might like to reconsider a point made in Chapter 3. I stated there my decision to use the word 'patient' because of its familiarity, but with the proviso that, because of its passive connotations, there is good reason for replacing it with the term 'client'. This chapter has underlined this, emphasizing the importance of handing over the locus of control to the patient, the practitioner acting as expert consultant rather than authoritarian dictator. A related point is the use of the phrase patient management: whether optometrists or psychologists, perhaps we should not think of ourselves as 'managing' patients, but as facilitators, creating the circumstances under which patients can better manage their own lives.

It is perhaps appropriate to leave the final word to Milder and Rubin (1978), who are not psychologists but ophthalmologists. To those who regard the psychological aspects of vision care as unnecessary, time-consuming hogwash they suggest, unapologetically, that they would be better employed in real estate or the fast-food industry. I sincerely hope that none of my readers is contemplating such a career change!

References

Allen J., Fraser K. (1983). Evaluation of visual capacity in visually impaired and multi-handicapped children. *Rehabil. Optom.*, **1**, 5.

Anderson B., Palmore E. (1974). Longitudinal evaluation of ocular findings. In *Normal Aging* (Palmore E., ed.). Durham, NC: Duke University Press.

Bandura A. (1977). Self-efficacy: toward a unifying theory of behaviour change. *Psychol. Rev.*, **84**, 191–215.

Barraga N. (1976). *Visual Handicaps and Learning: A Developmental Approach*. Belmont, California: Wadsworth.

Birren J.E., Williams M.V. (1982). A perspective on aging and visual function. In *Aging and Human Visual Function* (Kline D., Sekule R., Dismukes K., eds). New York: Alan R. Liss.

Carson G. (1990). Psychological factors in physical disability: a study investigating stress and emotions in people with significant physical disabilities. Paper given to Scottish Branch of British Psychological Society, Perth, September, 1990.

Chapman E.K., Stone J.M. (1988). *The Visually Handicapped Child in Your Classroom*. London: Cassell.

Coupland N., Giles H., Benn W. (1986). Language, communication and the blind. *J. Lang. Soc. Psychol.*, 53–64.

Dodds A.G. (1988). *Mobility Training for Visually Handicapped People: A Person-centred Approach*. London: Croom Helm.

Dodds A.G. (1989). Motivation reconsidered: the importance of self-efficacy in rehabilitation. *Br. J. Visual Impairment*, **VII**, 11–15.

Faye E., Padula W., Padula J. et al. (1984). The low vision child. In *Clinical Low Vision* (Faye E.E., ed.). Boston: Little, Brown.

Ferrell K.A. (1984). The editors talk. . .(guest editorial). *Ed. Visually Handicapped*, **16**, 43–6.

Fraiberg S. (1977). *Insights from the Blind. Comparative Studies of Blind and Sighted Infants*. New York: Basic Books.

Gardner A., McCormack A. (1990). The potential role of communication in developing self efficacy in the patient. Paper presented to 5th European Regional Conference of Rehabilitation International, Dublin, Ireland.

Genensky S.M. (1976). Acuity measurements—do they indicate how well a partially sighted person functions or could function? *Am. J. Optom. Physiol. Opt.*, **53**, 809–12.

Hill J.L. (1987). Rights of low vision children and their parents. *Can. J. Optom.*, **49**, 78–83.

Hofstetter H.W. (1985). Unmet vision care needs. *J. Vision Rehabil.*, **3**, 16.

Kirchner C., Peterson R. (1979). The latest data on visual disability from NCHS. *Visual Impairment Blindness*, April, 151–3.

Kirchner C., Philips B. (1980). Report of a survey of U.S. low vision services. *J. Visual Impairment Blindness*, **74**, 122–4.

Kobasa S.C. (1979). Stressful life events, personality and health: an enquiry into hardiness. *J. Pers. Soc. Psychol.*, **37**, 1–11.

Kobasa S.C.O., Pucetti M.C. (1983). Personality and social resources in stress resistance. *J. Pers. Soc. Psychol.*, **45**, 839–50.

Kolata G. (1986). Blindness of prematurity unexplained. *Science*, **231**, 20–2.

Kubler-Ross E. (1969). *On Death and Dying*. New York: Macmillan.

Leat S.J., Karadsheh S. (1991). Use and non-use of low vision aids by visually impaired children. *Ophthalmic Physiol. Opt.*, **11**, 10–15.

Leat S.J., Rumney N.J. (1990). The experience of a university-based low vision clinic. *Ophthalmic Physiol. Opt.*, **10**, 8–15.

Leung E., Hollins M. (1989). The blind child. In *Understanding Blindness* (Hollins M., ed.). New Jersey: Lawrence Erlbaum.

Lindstedt E. (1986). Early vision assessment in visually impaired children at TRC, Sweden. *Br. J. Visual Impairment*, **IV**, 49–51.

Lovie-Kitchin J. E., Bowman K.J. (1985). *Senile Macular Degeneration*. Boston: Butterworths.

Milder B., Rubin M.L. (1978). *The Fine Art of Prescribing Glasses Without Making a Spectacle of Yourself*. Florida: Triad.

O'Malley T.P., Newmark T.S., Rothman M.I., Strassman M.D. (1989). Emotional aspects of cataract surgery. *Int. J. Psychiatry Med.*, **19**, 85–9.

Padula W.V. (1982). Low vision related to function and service delivery for the elderly. In *Aging and Human Visual Function* (Kline D., Sekuler R., Dismukes K., eds). New York: Alan R. Liss.

Robbins H.G., McMurray N.E. (1988). Psychological and visual factors in low vision rehabilitation of patients with age related maculopathy. *J. Vision Rehabil.*, **2**, 11–21.

Seligman M.E.P. (1975). *Helplessness: On Depression, Development and Death*. San Fransisco: Freeman.

Shindell S. (1988). Psychological sequelae to diabetic retinopathy. *J. Am. Optom. Assoc.*, **59**, 870–4.

Snyder L.H., Pyrek J., Smith K.A. (1976). Vision and mental function of the elderly. *Gerontologist*, **16**, 491–5.

Tobin M.J., Hill E.W. (1987). Special and mainstream schooling. Some teenagers' views. *New Beacon*, **LXXI**, 3–6.

Tobin M.J., Hill E.W. (1988). Visually impaired teenagers: ambitions, attitudes, and interests. *J. Visual Impairment Blindness*, **82**, 414–16.

Tobin M.J., Hill E.H. (1989). The present and future: concerns of visually impaired teenagers. *Br. J. Visual Impairment*, **VII**, 55–7.

Tuttle D.S. (1984). *Self-esteem and Adjusting with Blindness: The Process of Responding to Life's Demands*. Springfield, Illinois: Charles. C. Thomas.

Index